# Contents

# Key messages

## The problems

- Acutely ill medical patients account for a high proportion of the inpatient work of NHS hospitals. These patients are usually admitted on an unplanned basis, often with complex needs that are difficult to diagnose.

- Care for acutely ill medical patients is delivered by teams of clinicians, including doctors from different specialties. These teams require information about patients' medical histories and test results that may not be readily available.

- Consultants responsible for these patients are usually not in contact with the patients' GPs. These consultants may also encounter difficulties in communicating with other consultants within their hospital and with colleagues in transferring hospitals.

- Providing safe and high-quality care to these patients has always been challenging but has become more so as the volume and complexity of work has increased. Clinical teams have absorbed growing pressures on the NHS but this is unlikely to be sustainable.

- Increases in the numbers of doctors, nurses, allied health professionals (AHPs) and other staff in hospitals have helped the NHS meet rising demand but there are now difficulties in filling vacancies. The use of agency staff to address workforce shortages has affected teamworking and continuity of care.

- Changes in medical training have also affected continuity of care and have resulted in a more fragmented and unsatisfactory experience for junior doctors, who comprise a core part of the clinical workforce.

## The solutions

- NHS organisations have adopted a variety of solutions to these problems. They include joining up disparate information systems, using board rounds alongside ward rounds to improve teamworking, improving handovers between nursing shifts, and understanding how patients experience care.

- Some trusts have adopted quality improvement programmes to find solutions, though the health care sector in England has generally been slow to do so and the number of organisations making a serious and sustained strategic commitment to quality improvement remains small.

- Some solutions aim to reduce unwarranted variations in how clinical care is provided to acutely ill medical patients by standardising the organisation of care on hospital wards. This may include specifying the composition of teams, interdisciplinary collaboration, and early treatment of the deteriorating patient.

- The Royal College of Physicians' Future Hospital programme is working with several hospitals to support improvements in care for acutely ill medical patients. The RCP is also supporting quality improvement work in acute medicine.

- The new care models programme is supporting hospitals to work more closely with general practices, community services and social care to develop whole-system solutions. The programme recognises that more fundamental improvements in the organisation of care are needed than are feasible within hospitals alone, including strengthening relationships between specialists and GPs.

## Priorities for the future

- The primary responsibility for delivering safe and high-quality care rests with the clinical teams that are providing care; trust leaders and national regulators are the second and third lines of defence respectively.

- Trust leaders should support clinical teams and managers by providing the training, resources and time they need to improve care. They should also themselves visibly attend to how care is organised at the front line and signal that this is an organisational priority.

- Leaders should value and trust staff, create the headroom for clinical teams to improve care, and seek and act on patient feedback. They should make it easy for staff to speak up without fear about the problems affecting the safety and quality of care.

- Clinical leaders have a key responsibility within trusts to connect clinical teams with trust leaders and jointly develop more effective ways of organising care on hospital wards and clinics.

- Leaders at all levels should focus on the operational aspects of how work is done in hospitals. They should remain in close touch with day-to-day work on clinical units and provide visible support to clinical teams.

- Action is urgently needed to improve the working lives of junior doctors and to seek and act on their insights into how care is organised and how it can be improved

- Regulators should provide the resources to modernise physical spaces, equipment and information technology, and to train and develop the workforce of the future.

- Regulators should also replace external support provided by management consultants with a commitment to quality improvement led by trust leaders with a track record of delivering change.

- Professional societies should build on the efforts of the Royal College of Physicians and use their resources and influence to support quality improvement work.

- Government has a responsibility to provide sufficient and sustainable funding to enable staff to meet rising patient demands safely and effectively.

#  Introduction

### Setting the scene: Chris Ham and Don Berwick

The idea for this report originated in two visits we made to Worthing Hospital during 2016 to see for ourselves the work being done to improve the quality of care for patients. During both visits we met the chief executive, Marianne Griffiths, and members of her senior team. We also visited different parts of the hospital to meet staff and see examples of how they are working to improve the services for which they are responsible. Here we describe what we saw and learnt.

### An outstanding trust

Every improvement journey has a back story and Worthing Hospital is no exception. It merged with St Richard's Hospital in Chichester in 2009 following an acrimonious debate about the reconfiguration of acute hospital services in West Sussex. The new leadership team focused initially on eliminating a combined deficit of £21 million, tackling an elevated hospital standardised mortality ratio (HSMR) of 115, and cutting long waiting times for treatment. The team then worked to become a foundation trust, achieving that status in 2013.

At around this time the senior team at the Western Sussex Hospitals NHS Foundation Trust, as it became known, heard about a model for improving patient safety at the Virginia Mason Medical Center (VMMC) in Seattle. Marianne Griffiths visited VMMC with colleagues to find out more about its approach to safety and improvement; she described being 'blown away' by what she learnt. The team also visited Salford Royal NHS Foundation Trust to understand how an NHS organisation was seeking to improve quality.

The upshot was a decision to establish the Patients First programme, which seeks to strengthen staff engagement and commitment to improvement through training and mentoring, with a particular focus on developing clinical leaders. In doing so the senior team at the trust drew on the experience of the Thedacare Centre for Healthcare Value, an organisation based in the United States that provides expertise to health care organisations committed to quality improvement. The trust's board provided funding of almost £2 million to support this work.

Patients First started in earnest in April 2015. As described by the medical director, George Findlay, the programme has five pillars:

- a series of improvement projects in areas including outpatients, endoscopy and operating theatres

- capability building among staff by providing training in lean methodologies to raise awareness of and skills in quality improvement

- the establishment of a 'kaizen office' staffed by six people with master black belt qualifications hired from outside the trust. (Kaizen is a Japanese word that means 'change for better' and is the practice of continuous improvement).

- strategic deployment encompassing sustainability, people, patient experience and quality objectives

- the 'Patients First Improvement System', which entails ward-based education for staff drawing on the expertise of Thedacare and staff in the kaizen office.

The results are evident in reductions in the HSMR (from 115 to 89) and in a wide range of innovations throughout the hospital. One of the most ambitious and impressive is a newly designed emergency floor that brings together the acute medical unit, the acute surgical unit and the acute frailty unit, alongside a clinical decision unit for patients about to breach the four-hour accident and emergency (A&E) target. The variety of resources available on the emergency floor, and the ways in which they are used, help explain the trust's consistently good performance on the A&E target.

In 2016 Western Sussex Hospitals NHS Foundation Trust was rated as 'outstanding' by the Care Quality Commission (CQC), which found much to admire there, including strong alignment between the leadership and ward staff around the goals and methods of Patients First. This reflects the investment made in staff engagement, continuity of leadership in the trust, the commitment to the development of clinical leadership and, above all, a culture committed to safety and quality as the organising principle. During our visits, we independently witnessed staff meeting in improvement huddles to review progress on their quality objectives and to engage in real-time problem solving.

Marianne Griffiths and her colleagues readily acknowledge that Patients First is a work in progress and not all parts of the hospital have yet been engaged. Nevertheless, it was clear to us that much has been achieved in a relatively short period of time, certainly when compared with other organisations going through a similar process of change and improvement. As Marianne explained to us, one of the lessons from VMMC was the need to exercise 'strategic patience' when embarking on a quality improvement journey, aiming for the accumulation of numerous marginal gains rather than a sudden breakthrough in performance.

Evidence of progress can be found in the trust's financial and operational performance, as well as in the CQC's assessment. At a time when most acute hospital providers are in deficit, Western Sussex continues to deliver a surplus and to hit most of its waiting time targets. The prospects are undoubtedly challenging but for now, at least, the trust has been able to buck the trend of declining performance evident in other parts of the NHS.

## The experience of frontline clinicians

During our visits, we had the opportunity to meet with Gordon Caldwell, a general physician who has worked at Worthing Hospital since 1993. Gordon is a longstanding champion of quality improvement methods and has pioneered the use of a ward round checklist in his practice. We each shadowed him on one of his ward rounds to gain some understanding of the experience of frontline clinicians working at the sharp end of acute medicine.

Before the ward round started we observed Gordon checking details on his office computer of the patients he would be seeing and we then accompanied him and his trainees as they visited these patients on a medical ward with 24 patients organised in six-bed bays. Patients were typically old and frail with multiple medical needs. There were three toilets on the ward and no space for staff to meet without interruption to review patients before the ward round.

Patients had little or no privacy during the ward round and discussions about patients were audible to those in adjacent beds. We observed the time it took to access patients' records, track down and interpret test results, and some of the challenges of communication between clinicians inside and outside the hospital. Subsequent to our visits, Gordon provided us with examples of patients he had cared for where concerns had arisen about the quality of their care.

One such patient was a 66-year-old man admitted to hospital from the A&E department with severe joint pains. Although it was known that the patient was under treatment for cancer at a nearby specialty hospital, neither Gordon nor his registrar was able to determine his chemotherapy regimen, which oncologists had treated him, or even with certainty whether he had been given antibiotics in A&E. The patient's GP had no information about his cancer centre treatment, and the admitting papers misidentified the type of cancer for which he was being treated.

A full week passed before the registrar was able to make contact with the treating oncologist, during which time the patient was treated, needlessly as it turned out, for a possible infection rather than for the cancer therapy reaction that was the true cause of his joint pain. The patient's entire course of treatment was confounded by misinformation, missing information and constant duplication, consuming the scarce time of the registrars and Gordon, not to mention presenting risks to the patient's wellbeing and ultimate outcome. Gordon later wrote: '[This patient's] case did not strike me as unusual or particularly remarkable. We are often left hunting around in the dark for vitally important facts about a patient's clinical condition.'

Gordon's experience and the experience of some of his patients draws attention to the difficulties facing frontline clinicians in providing the best possible care in the NHS – even in well-led organisations like Western Sussex with a deep commitment to quality improvement, and with results to demonstrate what has been achieved. Our summary of these difficulties, in no particular order, is as follows.

- Staff working under constant pressure (notwithstanding substantial increases in staffing in recent years) in the face of growing demand from an ageing population with complex needs.

- Difficulties in communicating with GPs about their patients who are admitted to hospital, including knowing who the GPs are for specific patients.

- Problems in communication within the hospital between acute medical staff and A&E staff as well as between different specialist teams.

- Difficulties in communicating with staff in other hospitals when patients are transferred.

- Delays in ordering and receiving the results of diagnostic tests, which in turn lead to delays in treatment and increases the time patients spend in hospital.

- Challenges in teamworking, for example on ward rounds when consultants might not be accompanied by trainees and nurses.

- Information systems that do not link data about patients held in primary and secondary care and that are often time consuming to use.

- Patients having to repeat their histories (where they are able to) at different stages in their treatment.

- Care being delivered inefficiently and often ineffectively because of the amount of duplication involved in all the above activites.

- Old buildings and cramped layouts that do not allow privacy and sometimes dignity for patients or space for staff to work without interruption.

- Disorganisation of supplies and workflows on clinical units.

Our initial reaction was that these difficulties signalled a 'disconnect' between frontline clinicians and the trust's senior leadership.

As we explored further, we realised this reaction was an oversimplification. The senior team is well aware of the frustrations encountered by clinicians in their daily work, and equally conscious that some of the causes, such as old buildings and disconnected information systems, are not within the trust's power to address, at least in the short term. The senior team is therefore focusing its efforts on those aspects of care that it can improve by working with frontline clinicians and by providing them with the skills and support to remove some of the barriers facing them.

### Is Worthing Hospital unusual?

In the course of our work, we found published studies that confirmed many of the observations we made in Worthing, most notably a paper in the *British Medical Journal* (*BMJ*) drawing attention to the particular challenges that arise in acute medicine (Pannick *et al* 2016b). As the paper notes, medical wards of the kind we visited deliver the majority of inpatient medical care in health systems worldwide and the workload on these wards involves 'treating complex, increasingly frail patients in a time pressurised setting'. The authors add:

> *Medical ward teams care for a particularly heterogeneous group of patients, with no single best pathway for diagnosis or treatment. Staff are skilled in the management of a diverse range of conditions, from pyelonephritis to gastrointestinal bleeding and terminal cancer. Many patients arrive without a diagnosis; indeed, empirical treatment can be concluded with no definitive diagnosis ever established.*

They continue:

> *Episodes of medical ward care can be long, involving large, dynamic, multidisciplinary teams. Team members are often dispersed throughout the hospital; physicians and allied health professionals are rarely located together on one unit with nurses and their patients. Frequent handovers are made more difficult by the absence of a central procedure around which a structured care narrative can be formed.*

> *Errors are common and often serious – medical ward patients have the same risks of preventable and fatal adverse events as those in intensive care and preventable hospital deaths are disproportionately caused by failures in general ward care. Crucially, ward failures are different from the procedural misadventures of the operating theatre or intensive care unit, resulting instead from the accumulation of missed opportunities to provide needed care.*

We have quoted at some length from this paper because it resonates strongly with much of what we saw and learnt on our visits. Pannick and colleagues outline four strategies to manage the complexity of care on acute medical wards, namely to standardise predictable care tasks to reduce specific harms; to simplify the care environment and the systems that support care delivery; to optimise effectiveness of interdisciplinary teams; and to engage patients in transitions of care. We return to discuss these and other ways of improving care at the front line in subsequent contributions to this report, including one from Sam Pannick.

## Insights from a roundtable

Further confirmation that Worthing Hospital is not unusual came from two roundtable discussions we convened at The King's Fund bringing together a number of people with different perspectives on these issues. Participants included junior and senior doctors from general medicine, general practice, the care of older people and other specialties, as well as experts in quality improvement and the chief inspector of hospitals from the CQC. Also involved were representatives of some of the medical royal colleges, which we consider important given their role in promoting high standards of medical care.

We were conscious that those of us who spend our lives working in or alongside the NHS are always at risk of accepting how care is delivered, defects and all, even when we may know that there is scope for improvement. A number of those at the roundtables, Don Berwick among them, helped illuminate how NHS practices compare with those in other systems, cautioning against either complacency or resignation. We challenged ourselves by asking whether the NHS has normalised standards and processes that might be seen as less acceptable in other countries.

In convening the roundtables, we wanted to check our observations at Western Sussex against the experience of colleagues from other hospitals. The discussion confirmed that the difficulties we had observed were not unique to Worthing Hospital. It also revealed that the delivery of acute medical care varies between hospitals. Aspects of the care we observed had been tackled successfully elsewhere by general physicians, geriatricians and others involved in the care of medical patients with complex needs. The essays in this report provide examples of where this is being done.

Some of those who took part urged us to avoid overcomplicating the analysis of what we saw and urged us to keep a practical focus on the core processes on acute medical wards that most lend themselves to improvement. Much of the discussion focused on the importance of relationships within and between clinical teams, and the cultures that support or hinder teamwork in the delivery of care. The NHS has often been described as a collection of professional tribes, each of which may find it difficult to rise above its own loyalties and work collaboratively with others to meet the needs of patients.

A key issue in teamworking is the role of doctors in training and the part they play in clinical care. It was noted that trainees often have observations and insights that can be of great value in understanding barriers to effective work and in constructing solutions. This is because they are less socialised into 'the way things are done around here', and because during training they have the benefit of observing and providing care in different hospitals. Finding ways of empowering trainees to contribute their observations on improving care was identified as one way of making progress.

A more general insight was the need to 'go to the gemba' and listen carefully to the ideas and experiences of all staff in order to fully understand safety and quality issues. Gemba is a Japanese word often used in work on quality improvement to denote the place where work is done – in this case the acute medical ward. This poses a challenge for The King's Fund because much of our work focuses on the policy context in which care is delivered and the organisational and system leadership needed to provide care of the highest possible standards within available resources. Our recent work has not explored the realities of care on the front line in any depth.

It is, however, a challenge we welcome for the opportunity it provides to understand better the relationship between national policies, local factors like the leadership of trusts, and frontline clinical care. The experience of patients is shaped by the interaction of all of these variables, including the funding made available by government, the way in which care is paid for within the NHS, how the quality of care is regulated, and the number and mix of staff delivering care. As the CQC has shown in its work, the quality of leadership of trusts and the engagement of staff are also important influences (Care Quality Commission 2017).

## This report

With these considerations in mind, we commissioned a series of essays from participants at the roundtables and others with experience of the realities of frontline clinical care. The report that follows brings together those essays, each written on aspects of the questions raised by our visits to Worthing Hospital. They enable readers to listen to the voices of staff and patients and are intended as the first contribution to an ongoing appreciative inquiry into care processes that are often imperfectly understood by policy-makers and senior health care leaders. Where relevant, we draw on the work of other researchers who have explored some of these issues from different perspectives (for example, Pannick *et al* 2016b and Bohmer 2009).

Most of the contributions to this report focus on the experiences of acutely ill medical patients in hospitals. These patients account for a high proportion of the work of acute hospitals and improving their experience of care has the potential to make a major difference to the challenges faced by frontline staff and the functioning of hospitals. They may be cared for on general medical wards, acute medical units, and wards and units specialising in the care of older people and frailty. Other areas of NHS care, including general practice and community nursing, face similar challenges but we have been unable to investigate them within the scope of our current appreciative inquiry.

One of the aims of this report is to begin a conversation about where responsibility should lie for mitigating and overcoming the difficulties we observed. One school of thought holds that the organisation of the English NHS creates an expectation that ministers or the Department of Health should intervene to improve care, following Bevan's famous dictum that when the bedpan falls to the floor in Tredegar Hospital, the sound should reverberate in the Palace of Westminster. This expectation has been reinforced by growing scrutiny and regulation on the part of national bodies like CQC in recent years and the erosion of promised autonomy for NHS bodies at a local level.

Another school of thought argues that responsibility for the provision of safe and high-quality care rests primarily with local leaders, both clinical and managerial. This view recognises that centralised decision-making and national regulation will always have a part to play in a health service funded through taxes and accountable via ministers to parliament. However, it contends that this should not obscure the responsibilities of others, including frontline clinicians, the leaders of NHS trusts and professional societies, for leading the design and redesign of more reliable systems to support care.

We start from the view that in a health care system like the NHS in which the reach of national bodies into frontline clinical care is tenuous and intermittent, those closest to where care is provided are usually best placed to make improvements. According to this view, a modern definition of professionalism assumes that frontline clinicians should seek and accept responsibility for identifying and removing obstacles to the delivery of high-quality care, with the support of others. We saw impressive evidence of this local commitment to improving care at Worthing Hospital, where clinical staff in many parts of the hospital were deeply engaged in process redesign as part of Patients First. We are aware that a number of other NHS hospitals are doing the same, as is reflected in some of the contributions that follow.

We hope and intend that this report and subsequent work will clarify the nature and extent of the need for better processes at the sharp end of NHS acute care. Even more, we hope to develop a shared view of the best balance between central oversight and regulation of care processes, and local and professionally led actions to improve patient outcomes and experiences. We return to reflect on these issues in our conclusion.

#  How is clinical care provided now?

## A physician's perspective: Elin Roddy

*Elin Roddy is a respiratory and general physician at Royal Shrewsbury Hospital and is lead clinician for smoking cessation, lung cancer and end-of-life care at the Shrewsbury and Telford Hospitals NHS Trust. She also sits on the Mortality and Morbidity Group and on the Local Negotiating Committee at the trust.*

It's 5.30pm on a winter Monday, already dark outside. On the way back from clinic, I take my customary detour up to the ward via the emergency department and the acute medical unit. If any of my patients are there, I like to know, and I also get to see what's happening around the hospital as I walk and talk.

In the emergency department, four patients wait in the corridor with ambulance crews. One lady is on oxygen, one on a drip, and there is a young patient under a blanket. The crews look weary, resigned to a wait. These are the same crews that should be responding to 999 calls but instead are trapped in a stuffy corridor waiting to hand over patients to staff who are overloaded and into beds that do not exist.

The emergency department board is a mix of red and black – red is bad, but black is worse. The colours signify how long patients have waited to be seen and sorted out. Many of the annotations read 'MBR' – medical bed requested – meaning patients have been seen and assessed, but there are no beds for them. But the waits to see emergency department doctors are also long. The junior doctors here are under pressure, and the senior and middle grade staff in the department are already working a ridiculous rota just to keep things safe. Locums cover gaps in rotas. There's nothing in the tank.

'What's the code for the gas machine?' someone in scrubs asks. 'Are you one of our doctors?' says the receptionist. 'I think so!' he says.

I cut through resus [resuscitation] to the acute medical unit. There are three patients in resus – a lady with a fractured hip, a febrile child and the patient who has just had the blood gas sample taken and who looks really sick. The junior doctor assessing him looks flustered and can't get hold of the medical registrar. There isn't one on duty until 9pm, I tell him. The day registrar had to go home to sleep in preparation to cover the night shift because the locum dropped out at the last minute. I look at the gas result and give some advice.

Through the door at the end of resus, I turn right into the acute medical unit doctors' office. Although it is only 5.30pm, the admissions board is almost full, and the second board will need to be started before the night shift come on – a bad sign. Many of the admissions are coming from the overstretched community teams, but there's also a high number from the emergency department. The early warning scores are written next to the names of each admission so that the team can prioritise the sickest patients.

The list of patients who have not yet been seen by a doctor is long, as the team is a doctor down today because of a rota gap, as well as missing a registrar. A cardiac arrest on another ward has taken the whole team out of action for the preceding 20 minutes, and they are just discussing how they will catch up. The consultant on call gives me a weary wave. He is trying to teach some medical students but keeps getting interrupted.

Round the corner, at the nurses' station, a conversation is taking place between the ward co-ordinator and the site manager about which escalation areas to open up overnight, and how they will be staffed. Another nurse is on the phone to my respiratory ward. She's trying to get hold of a nurse there to hand a patient over in order to free up a bed on the acute medical unit (AMU) for one of the patients in the emergency department. I'd like the man in resus to go straight to my ward, but he hasn't been waiting long enough.

An occupational therapist is on another phone. 'I'd like to speak to the duty social worker please, urgently.' We no longer have hospital social workers, so getting non-medical issues sorted is really tricky. There's a possible safeguarding problem, and urgent care is required for a relative. But home care is almost impossible at the moment, and waits are long, meaning patients are stranded in hospital. A relative approaches the desk: 'I've been waiting here for an hour to talk to someone about my father.' I apologise and find the nurse in that bay to give him an update. She is doing the drug round; I am not supposed to interrupt her but I do. It might make a medication error more likely, but may avoid a complaint.

I head past the AMU kitchen and down through ambulatory care, where nine or ten patients wait in a cramped reception area. One or two are clearly going to need admitting into beds, but there are no empty beds and they are relatively safe here – at least until the nursing staff finishes at 9pm. There is a backlog in assessing these patients because of a lack of rooms, and the doctors keep being bleeped away. There's nowhere for the staff to write notes, and very little privacy. It's hot. There's a sign on the exit door telling people not to use it as a short cut. I take a short cut through it onto the corridor.

Up on the respiratory ward there are two patients sat out by the nurses' station eating their tea while waiting for transport. One bed is ready for the next patient, but the nurses haven't had a chance to take handover [information sharing about a transferred patient]. The other bed space needs cleaning but it's tea-time and there is no housekeeper today so the health care assistants are giving out the meals first. Four patients of mine are 'medically fit' to go home, and would be safer there, but need their care assessments completing first. The form is several pages long, and has to be assessed by an external social worker to see what care and support will be funded.

I am asked by one of the physiotherapists to look at a man with pneumonia who is on a high-flow humidified oxygen Airvo device, and then I call in to see one of my patients in a side room who is dying of lung cancer. He is agitated, his son is upset and I find the nurse looking after him to ask for some more midazolam. She is in the middle of a drug round and the other nurse is not signed off for controlled drugs yet, so I know there is going to be a delay in him getting the medication. I wonder if a syringe driver might be better, to avoid these delays, but then worry that he would not be alert enough to talk to his daughter who is due to arrive tonight from London.

I sit at the desk on the ward to write up some meds and answer the phone five or six times. Most of the calls are from relatives wanting updates, or from AMU wanting to give handover.

I try to stall them on AMU, because I want my patient to get his midazolam, but I also want the chap in resus to get a bed. One of the relatives who phones is someone I need to speak to anyway, and we make a very straightforward resuscitation decision and escalation plan together over the phone.

This all takes around 30 minutes. I see many tiny kindnesses on my travels. I see lots of patients getting good and compassionate care, and I see lots of colleagues bending over backwards to ensure that things get done. I see lots of patients and families waiting patiently, knowing that we are doing our best, thanking the staff for their hard work. And our hospital is not unique. These scenes are being played out up and down the country.

But sometimes we don't – can't – notice them. We have made ourselves so used to this new 'normal' that noticing it all – the sub-optimal processes, the unnecessary delays, the broken promises – would make it impossible to come to work. They say that 'the standard you walk past is the standard you accept'. I don't accept these things that I see – people on trolleys in corridors, patients waiting for vital medication, families in distress. These things are not acceptable. We should not walk past.

But if everybody keeps stopping, who is going to do the work?

*This article first appeared as a blog at:* https://elinlowri.wordpress.com/2017/02/13/the-standard-you-walk-past-is-the-standard-you-accept/

### A trainee's perspective: Jennifer Isherwood

*Jennifer Isherwood is senior general surgical trainee in the Oxford region. She appreciates the need for doctors to take a more active role in management and leadership of the NHS and recognises the impact this can have on services, staff and most importantly patient care. Jennifer has taken a year out of training to develop her skills in and understanding of successful leadership and management.*

A trainee's day falls into one of two categories: emergency or elective work. Both follow a similar pattern: arrive, hand over, see patients (ward round and review new referrals), clinic/endoscopy/theatre, hand over, go home. As a rule of thumb, elective work is more predictable and controlled. Despite this, the 'nags' of the working day remain the same and although seeming simple are nowhere near resolution.

**Handover:** A universally recognised process of communication between the incoming and outgoing doctors, to relay information about which patients are unwell, which need review and which investigations should be chased. Like any meeting, the quality of a handover is dependent on the chair. In my view, there are three cardinal keys to success at any meeting or handover:

- be on time

- have a prepared list of patient details for all incoming doctors

- set a brief agenda at the start, ie, 'We have admitted X number of patients. There are Y number still to be seen and I am concerned about Z number of patients. We will discuss each in more detail.'

The latter two points rely on good team communication, informing a single, usually most junior, doctor about the required data to update the patient list.

This will unlock a Pandora's box of IT issues: finding a computer with connecting printer that works, having appropriate knowledge of the programme or Excel to create a well formatted list, and ensuring there is paper available to print the list. With the commencement of handover inevitably comes the bombardment of bleeps that interrupt discussions with conversations or requests that likely could have waited 30 minutes.

**Ward round:** Following handover the ward round begins. Led by the most senior member of the medical team, it follows this pattern: find patient, review notes and charts, consult with patient, agree management plan and repeat with next patient. It's a methodical ritual that underpins almost every aspect of a doctor's job.

### Step one – find your patient

Whether the patient was last seen five hours or five minutes ago, they will now have been moved. This triggers a frantic chicken-run of junior doctors trying to identify the correct nurse or ward clerk to update you with the patient's new location. If you're lucky the patient is still in the same ward so your planned ward round doesn't need to be re-routed; alternatively you back-track your movements because you unknowingly passed that patient in the corridor. All the while these tasks are knocking minutes off your working day – time that would be better spent talking to patients.

## Step two – find the notes

There are usually two sets of notes: nursing notes for observation charts, fluid balance tables, nutrition records etc. and medical notes for review documentation, printed investigation and correspondence. Logic would place these notes in their allocated position for the patient's bed number. This designated location varies between wards. The nursing staff handover is at a staggered time to the doctors' handover, so the nurses are now usually in the midst of their own reviews or medication rounds. They will have bundled the notes onto their trolley, guarding them like a new mother, because they too have just completed the marathon of identifying which patients they are responsible for and where their notes are.

## Step three – patient review

Having been the relative of a hospital patient, I question how patients maintain trust and a rapport with the medical profession. Modern shift patterns mean patients rarely see the same doctor more than once. Patients are repeatedly asked the same questions over and over. Gone are the days when a junior member of staff would clerk the patient, formulate a management plan more substantial than 'senior review', and then present their work to the lead clinician.

My heart sinks every time a patient asks, 'Isn't it in my notes?'. No patient wants to hear the woes about why their notes aren't shared between medical establishments locally or nationally and how as an organisation we struggle to find individual patients' notes, let alone record them chronologically. Attempts to contact other community or specialist teams can result in hours of missed calls and forgotten emails.

Communication breakdowns occur not just between hospitals and the outside world. No longer does the matron join the ward round and disseminate any decisions to her nursing staff. Workforce organisation limits co-joined work between nurses and the medical team.

Nurses' responsibilities limit their availability to join a medical ward round. Often multiple medical teams will work simultaneously, making it impossible for a nurse to be present on all of them at once. This stymies the flow of information between the nursing and medical staff and instead relies on the most junior member of the team finding the relevant nurse to inform them of any relevant management decision – cue the scurry of frantic chickens.

## Step four – action jobs

On completion of the ward round, the senior clinician will depart to attend to other clinical duties – eg, outpatients – leaving the frazzled junior doctors to action their management plans. Here starts the administration: liaising with other members of the multidisciplinary team, requesting tests and reviews and chasing their outcome. As the experience and autonomy of the junior doctors develop they may start to analyse and action results.

The biggest bugbear of most doctors' hospital lives is the computer system. Each doctor is armed with a plethora of logins, different for the fundamental IT programmes. The IT programmes used often differ between hospitals, which requires retraining and familiarisation every 6 to 12 months following the rotation of hospital sites. The processes for requesting investigations again change – some require discussion, some are on paper, others are all online.

Assuming you can find a rare gem – otherwise known as an available computer – you waste time trying combinations of your initials and names with varying passcodes to find the right combination to grant you access. Once in, you pray the system won't crash half way through what you are doing. It may or may not be connected to a printer, which may or may not have ink and paper (replacements of these are hidden in an unknown location). You don't dare depart this rare gem, once found, in case one of your colleagues, by now circling like birds of prey, start to use it or the computer logs you out.

Beware the kind doctor who attempts to rectify any of these issues by contacting IT helpdesk or looking to replenish depleted resources. This will lead you down a path of dead ends, long waits and bad on-hold music before you will invariably be given the advice, 'Have you tried turning it off and on again?' But don't worry; tomorrow you get to do it all again.

## A medical student's perspective: Harrison Carter

*Harrison Carter has co-chaired the British Medical Association's UK medical student committee since 2013. He is a Newton Masters Scholar at Downing College, Cambridge, completing a Masters in public health between the penultimate and final years of his medical degree at Bristol. He was a Lister Student at Oxford University.*

Medical students rotate through clinical placements in their final three years of study. The timetables at medical schools are tailored to ensure that medical students experience different hospital environments, from large tertiary and regional referral centres to district general hospitals. In addition to different hospital environments, medical students rotate around different medical, surgical and specialty teams.

During each rotation students will be assigned a consultant or senior doctor and will spend time shadowing the junior doctors. They will be encouraged to clerk patients, and to examine and carry out simple clinical skills, under supervision.

Medical students' perspectives are unique. They rotate around parts of a hospital where there may be low doctor turnover and so they could be the freshest pair of eyes present. Their observations may therefore challenge established ways of working in the sense that they, perhaps, become aware of deficient practices that others simply hadn't noticed.

Medical students are regarded as the most junior members of the team – if they are considered as part of the team at all. This is because they are not responsible for the provision of care (even if their actions have an impact on patients) and because they have not yet gained a primary medical qualification. So, although medical students could be the most able to identify poor practice or areas for improvement (through direct comparison with more recent clinical experience elsewhere), they lack the authoritative ability to highlight this to the appropriate people.

Medical students are much less able than any other member of the team to be independent change-makers themselves. This is largely because they lack 'process and procedures' knowledge.

### The issues

Junior doctors are ambitious and hard-working. Medical students, like myself, often see them as role models. In today's NHS, junior doctors find themselves stretched to cover rotas and often work well past the end of their shift in an attempt to provide the safest care for their patients. However, they are reluctant to raise overworking as an issue.

What seems to stop them is a 'learned helplessness'. With the NHS dominating headlines, this thought process of helplessness is seeping into medical schools and affecting medical students, prompting them to consider their place in the NHS. In medical school, I have observed the hidden curriculum, which could be acting as a barrier to innovation and the improvement of care.

Sometimes we observe that our more senior colleagues find it difficult to communicate with health care professionals outside the hospital. In primary care, we observe the same frustrations when general practitioners struggle to engage their hospital colleagues.

We listen to some of the language used to describe members of different medical and surgical specialties. We begin to form our own opinions – opinions which, in the future, risk perpetuating a culture that hinders teamwork and the seamless delivery of high-quality care.

As a student, I experience different ward environments every couple of weeks during regular rotations at medical school. In doing this, I compare how different wards address and solve safety and quality concerns. The differences between wards are as stark as the differences between hospitals and between trusts.

Medical students could contribute to the process of improving care. My view, for example, is that understanding how national policies are framed by local trust leadership and what impact that has on frontline care would be a first step in the right direction.

## The solutions

Thoughtful attention to these issues, away from the spotlight, may help us understand how we listen to each other and enable us to use frontline experiences to find solutions. Often, solutions that can be embedded into hospital practice are inexpensive, relatively simple and innovative.

The first is to consider how we work alongside those who want to modernise medical teaching and education. A greater emphasis could be placed on generalist skills. Medical students will need to be prepared to treat more complex, increasingly frail patients in a time-pressured setting. Making them aware of the 'barriers' and 'difficulties' that arise from providing this kind of care will allow students to develop their critical thinking and change their approach in future practice to overcome problems. They will become resilient practitioners.

I have observed how different members of the team will care, cure and prevent disease and disability in different ways. Some of the most valuable learning I have acquired has been from physiotherapists, nurses, midwives, speech and language and occupational therapists. In mental health services, social workers have been an invaluable source of experience and knowledge. A first exposure to the multidisciplinary team could come at medical school. Making this common practice would establish multidisciplinary working for the most junior members of the team once they have qualified.

Currently, the first experience of quality improvement for doctors is some years after qualification. While this is in no way tokenistic, their participation is often limited. Medical schools could consider running 'innovate local quality improvement' project competitions. I have seen first-hand medical students designing simple solutions to some of the problems that patients and families face in hospitals. Simple ideas like these could empower medical students to want to continue this work in the future.

### A GP perspective: Rammya Mathew and John Launer

*Rammya Mathew is an academic clinical fellow in general practice and is undertaking a National Medical Director's Clinical Leadership Fellowship. She is currently part of a team at the Royal College of Physicians that is setting up a quality improvement hub aimed at giving health care teams the skills to improve services locally.*

*John Launer is associate dean, multi-professional faculty development for London and the South East, Health Education England. He was a GP for more than 20 years and also is trained as a family psychotherapist. He is currently lead programme director for educational innovation at Health Education England, an honorary senior lecturer at University College London and honorary consultant at the Tavistock Clinic.*

GPs have considerable insight into the care that their patients receive as we are commonly the ones to instigate the acute admission. We also take over the ongoing care of our patients following hospital discharge and are therefore privy to the stories that patients tell of their hospital admissions. The following remarks are drawn from our own experiences, and from interviews we carried out with around ten GP colleagues in preparation for writing this contribution.

## Hospital care of patients

As one might expect, GPs hear accounts of exemplary care, but also many accounts of chaotic, disjointed care that falls short of patient and GP expectations. There is likely to be an entire spectrum in between, but patients probably don't comment so much when things go relatively smoothly and care is just about good enough.

Perhaps our most pertinent reflection is that the concept of holistic care is fast disappearing. Patients are often subjected to 'quick-fix' treatments, without a sense of anyone taking overall responsibility for their care needs. This is particularly concerning given the growing problem of multi-morbidity, but at the same time unsurprising given the increasing trend towards specialism and super-specialism. As a result, there appears to be a very real and evident gap in terms of what patients need and what hospital physicians are able to provide.

Hospital teams often overlook patients' circumstances and their ability to cope independently following hospital discharge. Older patients are sometimes discharged very late at night or at weekends, without appropriate follow-up plans in place and then are readmitted shortly afterwards. A failure to look beyond their medical needs and an inability to view the patient as a person is frequently at the heart of this.

GPs acknowledge that the hospital environment is not always conducive to providing person-centred care. We are aware that wards are overcrowded and noisy, staff overworked, and information about the patients' background sparse. These factors cumulatively contribute to a sense of 'firefighting', in which the clinicians sometimes struggle to provide safe medical care, let alone have the luxury of finding out what matters most to the person and addressing this.

## GP communication with hospitals

On speaking to our colleagues, there were mixed views about the ease of communication between primary and secondary care. The consensus is that communication is dependent on both systems and personalities – and that one of these cannot compensate for the other.

For GPs, it can be difficult to get through to hospital colleagues for advice and clarification. It is not always clear who the appropriate contact person is, and once that person has been reached there can be a lack of understanding about the GP's concerns. Many hospital doctors give the impression that their priority is to prevent admissions, and do not appear to be able to put themselves in the GP's shoes.

In our experience it is vanishingly rare to get a call from the local hospital team seeking information or advice about a patient. One colleague reported that she sometimes receives a flurry of calls inquiring about patients from foundation year doctors in their first week or two working in hospitals – but then never hears from any of them again. Our perception is that hospital teams are too busy.

Hospital colleagues often don't appreciate the wealth of information that we have as GPs. This not only takes the valuable form of the computerised GP record (which these days is generally far more comprehensive and organised than hospital records), but we also have 'knowledge of the person' – a less tangible but often essential part of good clinical decision-making.

The way in which GPs work has also changed. New GPs are commonly working part-time and engaging in portfolio careers, so the provision of continuity is not as strong as it used to be. The combination of these factors makes it all too easy for things to slip through the net when patients are transferred between care environments.

Virtually all the GPs we spoke to said that the speed and (in general) the standard of hospital discharge notes had improved. Also, when hospital doctors and GPs collaborate, it seems to be a positive experience for the clinicians involved and the patient. One colleague described doing a joint home visit with an elderly care consultant and commented: 'Brilliant – this is how things could work, it could have taken dozens of letters to sort out – but I've not seen her before or since.'

Likewise, we are increasingly using email as a source of advice from hospital specialists, and when this process works well it enables us to provide responsive care and sometimes to avoid unnecessary hospital referral/admission.

## Our conclusions

Our overall impression from reflecting on our own experiences and from talking to a selected group of colleagues is that patients' experiences of care on acute wards, and GPs' experiences of communication from hospital staff, are variable, unpredictable and unsystematic. We heard of some outstanding examples of care and communication, but also of many failures to inform – or elicit information from – patients or their GPs. While we did not form the view that the system is 'broken down' or dysfunctional as a whole, it is clear that there are no regular standards or practices for involving patients or GPs in care, either within individual hospitals or across the secondary sector.

## A physician's perspective: Gordon Caldwell

*Gordon Caldwell has been a consultant physician at Worthing Hospital since 1993. In 2009 he attended the International Forum on Quality and Safety in Healthcare, and decided to improve the service to patients on ward rounds. His work has focused on teamworking and the use of checklists to improve process and reliability.*

This is a story of tragic misdiagnosis. It demonstrates how weaknesses in inpatient clinical review systems can contribute to poor decisions being made.

The story begins with a patient's admission to hospital with breathlessness and swelling in one leg. On the sixth day after admission, the patient collapsed with a major pulmonary embolism. Despite treatment, the patient died the next day.

Before admission, a relative of the patient had noticed the swollen leg and breathlessness, and after searching on Google, wondered if the patient had a deep vein thrombosis (DVT) and a pulmonary embolism (PE). On arriving at hospital, the relative told a nurse in Accident and Emergency (A&E) of the concerns about DVT and PE.

For the time up to their collapse on the sixth day, however, the patient was treated for community-acquired pneumonia and only had a dose of Dalteparin used for prevention – not treatment – of DVT. The patient was reviewed on the second and fourth days by a ward round team led by a consultant in respiratory diseases and on the fifth day by a team led by myself, a consultant in general medicine.

With the benefit of time to study the case in detail, the patient had a definite but mild pneumonia and DVT and PE, but was treated only for pneumonia. In retrospect, the failings that I could identify in caring for this patient were as follows.

- The nurse in A&E did not inform the A&E doctor of the relative's concerns about DVT and PE.

- The admitting doctor in the acute medical unit did not identify the swollen leg.

- The chest x-ray and blood gases would indicate a high probability of PE, because the area of pneumonia was small, but the oxygen levels were very low and the patient was a non-smoker. On the very busy ward round it seems likely that the consultant in respiratory diseases was not shown the chest x-ray and gases simultaneously.

- On day four the patient was making progress, so the treatment for pneumonia appeared to be working.

- The day I took over the patient's care was very busy, and I accepted without deep questioning the diagnosis of the respiratory consultant. On the ward round the patient's chest was examined, but not his legs. Again, the patient was making progress as if the treatment for pneumonia was working.

There is all the time in the world to sift through the information and identify in retrospect where the errors began that eventually led to a fatal outcome. At the time, the consultant in respiratory diseases had 25 acute admissions to review and it was a Saturday morning with fewer consultants and junior doctors working compared to weekdays, so much more pressure on time. The consultant would have been working with a team of doctors, possibly including some he had never worked with before.

The room where case discussion took place was small, subject to constant interruption, and did not have a high definition monitor for reviewing chest x-rays. At the patient's bedside, the consultations would be hurried because of the need to get the night team away on time, and simply to battle through the 25 cases. Almost certainly there would have been no nurse present during the consultant review, perhaps to raise the concern about the swollen leg.

When the patient came under my care, we had 27 cases to see that morning, many new to us. Our work space was very cramped and again there was no high-definition monitor. We were under intense pressure from management to 'discharge as many as possible, as early as possible'.

I have used a story with a dramatically tragic outcome, but the weaknesses in structure and process for inpatient clinical review on ward rounds, in my experience, affect every inpatient clinical review. Good decisions during case presentation need good information. This needs to be provided in a way, and in physical and psychological environments, that free the clinicians' minds for clinical thinking prior to consulting with the patient.

At the bedside clinicians need access to the relevant information in a manner that is easy to assimilate. It needs to be easy to talk with and examine the patients, without feeling that this is a huge effort, and without feelings of being hurried, distracted and interrupted.

The relevant information for clinical review is usually hard to find, gather and present in a way that supports releasing the mind for clinical thinking. The commonest word in handovers is 'chase' as in 'chase the CT scan request', then 'chase the CT report' and so on. Clinicians in current NHS ward environments are 'hunter-gatherers' of information and our capacity for attention, clinical thinking and safe decision-making can be exhausted by the efforts required to hunt out and gather information that is usually there somewhere.

The information of most value to the doctor clerking (taking a patient's medical history and undertaking an examination), the patient and to the consultant reviewing the case includes:

- recent well-composed discharge summary or summaries

- recent well-composed clinic letter(s)

- a list from the GP's database of the patient's long-term conditions and important past medical events – eg, surgery for breast cancer eight years ago

- a list of the patient's current prescribed medications

- results of previous tests and investigations – eg, for a breathless patient, knowing the results of a previous echocardiogram, lung function tests and blood tests for blood count and kidney function are very helpful.

These five simple factors are currently not easily available for acute admissions. I know that similar challenges face doctors throughout NHS hospitals. Some organisations have far better IT links with primary care, making it easier to gather in the information.

There is a common theme here: supporting clinical consultations in a way that frees minds for clinical thinking, planning and communication is of paramount importance for getting correct diagnosis and correct treatment. If the diagnosis and treatment are incorrect, the outcomes cannot be optimal.

Is there a way ahead? One idea is to define what I call 'quality indicators' for clinical consultations. If we are to improve the outcomes of the clinical consultations we need some quality indicators to help gauge whether the consultations were optimal or defective. These are the indicators that I suggest as a starting point for discussion.

- The patient should be as prepared as possible.

- The clinician should be as prepared as possible.

- The clinician should know the person, before making the person into a patient.

- The consultation should feel unhurried to patient and clinician.

- The clinician should be able to give undivided attention to the patient.

- The clinician should be able to hear herself or himself think.

- The consultation should be supported by information presented clearly and comprehensibly.

- The consultation should ensure confidentiality and dignity.

- The clinician should be regularly refreshed.

- An 'important other' – a relative or a friend – should be encouraged, with the patient's permission, to participate in the consultation.

## A patient's perspective: Michael Wise

*Michael Wise was a specialist in both oral surgery and restorative dentistry. In January 2009, he contracted sepsis with near-fatal consequences. As a clinician he astutely observed the spiral of events that followed and has since published a book,* On the toss of a coin (*Wise 2017*), *about his experience.*

In January 2009, I was rapidly transformed from being very fit and healthy to almost dead in intensive care. I acquired sepsis, which developed into toxic shock, causing multi-organ failure. I was on life support and in a medically induced coma for 10 of the 14 days of my stay in intensive care. I was subsequently hospitalised for seven weeks and since I had stage III acute kidney injury, I then required dialysis for 14 months. I received a live donor kidney transplant in March 2010 and have since made a good recovery. During the dialysis period there was an acute admission for sepsis and another admission post-transplant for a severe infection.

Overall, the care that I have received from frontline staff, primarily from the NHS, has been outstanding. I therefore have some reservations about describing the adverse findings as reported below because I do not want to detract from this overall excellence of care. However, I think it is important to point out some of the shortcomings and possible solutions based on my observations.

### Developing trust

From a patient's perspective it is important to feel that clinicians have knowledge and expertise in their field but, in addition, the development of trust at all levels in the care chain is essential. As in all walks of life it can take time for trust to be established, but it can be very easily and rapidly lost. When trust is lost, the patient's experience is severely compromised.

The development of trust is facilitated by the efficient and correct use of procedures. To give a simple personal example, I had a cannula inserted for the administration of intravenous (IV) antibiotics. I knew that it was not positioned into a vein, but the nurse would not listen. I then had repeated IV infusions of antibiotic causing severe pain and swelling of my hand. It was only when I was seen later the next day by a consultant that the cannula was correctly placed. My trust in that nurse evaporated very rapidly. Patients do know when something is wrong and they should be listened to.

Trust is also very importantly generated by interpersonal relationships and communication. I was unconscious during most of my intensive care stay, but I understand that the intensive care staff were remarkably caring and compassionate to my family, explaining to them the meaning of tests, alarms and equipment readings, and giving them time. They rapidly gained the trust of my family who, of course, in their own way were also a part of the illness. Family and partners should be seen as such.

## Positive communication

In intensive care, although unconscious and unresponsive to external stimuli, I could hear many things that were said. One was that someone thought I had suffered a stroke. When I heard that, I switched off and decided to die. Apparently around this period the crash team was summoned and my family was called in to say goodbye. Fortunately, I subsequently heard someone say, 'He hasn't had a stroke' and I changed my mental attitude. It really highlights to me the importance of taking great care as to what is said across an unconscious and/or sedated patient. In fact, it underlines the importance of taking great care with the use of language in general. Staff at all levels would benefit from role play regarding the use of language.

Six years after my transplant I was admitted to the same ward with a severe infection. I was saddened to see the obvious reduction in nursing staff and the unreasonable pressures placed on them. As a result, communication from some of the staff decreased. Non-verbal communications such as a smile, a touch or a reassuring squeeze of the hand, and verbal communication statements such as 'We are here to help you' or 'We've seen it all before' were frequently missing. Unfortunately, being busy can be used as an excuse for not being human, and there is a danger of this occurring among all frontline staff due to pressures. When feeling unwell, the negative interactions carry far more weight than the positive ones. I feel that it is important that the small aspects of communication are constantly reinforced to everybody in the medical chain, from consultants to tea trolley personnel.

Since the hospital is the medical and ancillary staff's working environment, it is very easy for them to become desensitised to the possible perspectives of patients. This can easily cause a deterioration of the patient's psychological health. Patients are frequently scared. They may be confused and anxious, but relieved to be cared for. However, the staff have no knowledge of any preconceived ideas that they bring with them when they enter hospital. The importance of small things should never be undervalued.

It seemed that when agency nurses were working on the ward, they frequently were not aware of the requirements of a transplant patient. There was great difficulty in obtaining water, and fluid levels were not adequately measured. These are basic requirements for all patients, but in particular for a transplant patient with a high temperature. I presume that similar situations may arise for other patients with special requirements.

The diagnosis and early treatment of acute kidney injury is an important issue across all acute medical services, particularly if this can reduce the estimate of up to 30,000 preventable hospital deaths per annum.

As an inpatient I was rarely informed of the order of the day and never informed as to how long it would take to get the results of tests. I suspect that this is a culture that could easily be reversed, though I acknowledge that some patients may not be able to absorb the information. Perhaps a checklist of the day's events given to patients would be helpful, but I appreciate this may create an enormous amount of additional work.

On some occasions large numbers of visitors were allowed into the ward to see one patient. When I was very ill, the bed next to me was surrounded by 14 visitors; in fact on one occasion it deteriorated into a fist fight between two of them. It was very unsettling. Control is essential, but perhaps the nurses simply do not have the time to manage such situations.

Bed blocking, of which as a patient I was very aware, is an obvious and highly publicised major problem and needs to be resolved urgently.

I must conclude as I started, by praising the overall level of care offered. It is vital that frontline clinical staff are valued, and told how much they are valued. They must not be made into scapegoats for the failings of an underfunded system, which needs to embrace digital technologies and which is greatly hampered by crumbling social care policies.

As a patient, it seems to be patently obvious that there is a limit to what a dedicated frontline workforce can do to improve the quality of care, or even to maintain it at its existing level. Further 'efficiencies' are likely to result in degradation of acute services, not improvement.

## A senior manager's perspective: Juliet Shavin

*Juliet Shavin is senior operations manager for medicine at the Royal Free London NHS Foundation Trust. During her 12 years with the Trust (previously Barnet & Chase Farm Hospital), Juliet has managed services in surgery, medicine and women's health. She has a Masters degree in occupational psychology and is an accredited performance coach.*

My team and I manage four services across two large acute hospitals and two smaller peripheral sites. Approximately 500 staff work in these sites and we provide both emergency and elective services to patients.

I love my job but trying to deliver world-class, affordable care every day in the current NHS environment is extremely challenging. The NHS and social care are under extraordinary financial pressure with a large funding gap, which influences almost every decision we make as a team. Balancing patient experience, outcomes and safety within this financial climate means my priorities are constantly changing.

In acute services, world-class care sometimes feels like it is defined nationally by targets. These targets include compliance with the four-hour accident and emergency (A&E) access target, the two-week wait for GP cancer referrals, the 62-day cancer treatment targets, the 18-week referral-to-treatment target, financial savings achieved, and so on. Targets can be helpful in quantifying, focusing and prioritising resources, but they can also be distracting. It can be challenging to get different professional groups to work together to deliver these targets while also supporting them to prioritise patient safety.

It feels like a constant juggling act to meet ever-increasing demand on services while at the same time removing cost from our budget. On one day, I can attend meetings discussing what budget we are going to remove to deliver the financial savings required. The very next day, I can be pulled in to meetings discussing how I can guarantee additional staff to meet the targets that we are not delivering. These 'crises', which can be caused by a spike in patient demand, staff going off sick, or difficulty in recruiting to vacancies, often require an immediate response.

One of the things I find most difficult about my job is containing the enthusiasm of clinicians, nurses and other team members when they come with great ideas about how they want to expand their services. As a good case in point we recently appointed a newly qualified consultant, full of enthusiasm and new ideas and who had trained for many years to become an expert in a particular area. Having her join the department was a breath of fresh air and the services have grown under her fledgling leadership.

With growth comes cost and we are now at the point where there is no more money available. I can feel the consultant's frustration as I explain why we can't implement the newest, best thing, that at the moment expansion is unaffordable, and that we have to direct resources towards the most pressurised areas, even if they would not be our first choice in an ideal world. I feel a great responsibility to my teams to support them in delivering the services that they want to provide, and we're working hard to think differently.

### Fair and transparent processes

Transparency and consistency hold the key to delivering the patient flow required to meet the needs of a demanding emergency department. We have implemented board-round protocols that are predictable and occur daily at the same time, so that all members of the multidisciplinary team (MDT) can be present and plans for the patients can be made early in the day. The operational managers regularly join the teams on the board rounds, to support the process and provide a mechanism to escalate any delays or blockages in the patient pathway, which includes access to diagnostics and specialty opinions.

We provide a bleep for immediate access to operational managers if they are not available. This gives us a very good understanding of the day-to-day challenges faced on the wards and we can consider solutions within the context of the wider organisation. We also regularly challenge assumptions to ensure the clinical team has prompt access to the services it needs. We have access to three bed meetings a day where we can escalate any issues to senior decision-makers and all the departments that are represented there.

In a busy acute hospital, it is essential that every patient receives an early daily clinical review and that all areas are covered consistently. To ensure a fair and transparent process, daily ward and specialty cover is now published weekly on a 'schedule' that is planned for in advance and communicated widely. Annual leave is authorised only when adequate cover is available and any issues are highly visible.

As a non-clinician, I am completely dependent on the team to advise on the best way forward for patient care. But I have the advantage of being able to ask the 'stupid questions' and challenge the status quo, without any real agenda. I can often provide a neutral, unbiased opinion to help agree the objectives between the different professional groups. I work with them on their suggestions, operationalising them and communicating them to the wider environment. Where possible we can put in measures to see if these processes have the desired effect and we are constantly reviewing and refining them.

Sometimes pressures beyond our control, such as the patients being cared for outside of their specialty wards, and social care constraints, compromise the delivery of service. It is essential that consistent care is delivered despite these frustrations. In these challenging situations, my job is to provide encouragement, support and a reminder of progress made. When things do not go as planned there is a great temptation for the organisation to apportion blame or implement a rapid change. It is my role to understand the difference between special and common cause variation and to apply the appropriate solution, challenging undesirable behaviours and protecting hard-working staff.

There are two areas where I think opportunities are available to the NHS. The first one – and when I worked in the private sector the easiest for quick wins – would involve employing IT solutions to automate monotonous non-value-added tasks. Fit-for-purpose IT systems would benefit the whole multidisciplinary team with one set of standardised, relevant patient information, to help save time and support safe decision-making.

The second is for us to be more comfortable with a culture of challenging our practice, constantly asking ourselves is this the best way, is this absolutely necessary. My favourite question to ask is: 'If I were the patient, would I want this appointment, test, or whatever, if it weren't absolutely necessary…' It is only then that we can really take waste out of the system and find the money to reinvest in new ways of doing things.

## A hospital manager's perspective: James O'Brien

*James O'Brien undertook the NHS graduate management training scheme and has held management roles at several trusts. He is currently at Guy's and St Thomas' NHS Foundation Trust where he is General Manager for Medicine and Neonatology at Evelina London Children's Hospital. In 2015 he co-launched the trust's management training scheme, which is about to recruit its third cohort of aspiring NHS managers. James has Masters in health and public leadership from the universities of Birmingham and Manchester.*

At Evelina London Children's Hospital, part of Guy's and St Thomas' NHS Foundation Trust, we have achieved great success in meeting demand even though resources are constrained. More patients are treated in all hospital settings than ever before. There are shorter lengths of stay in all but the most complex areas of care. More clinics and education are delivered in local district general hospitals, GP surgeries and child development centres in our local boroughs.

In spite of this progress, we find ourselves with more children attending and being admitted from accident and emergency (A&E) and the most inconsistent performance against the four-hour A&E target than we've ever had. Elective and diagnostic waiting times are increasing and we are admitting fewer children for urgent tertiary review from local hospitals than in previous years.

The constant balance of priorities between emergency department admissions and elective medical or surgical admission and inter-hospital patient transfer involves art, science and an increasing amount of prayer to the NHS gods.

An instance from a recent week on call highlights the gravity of these priorities.

It was 2pm and the hospital was full. Intensive care and high dependency were fully occupied; the emergency department was seeing an unusually early surge in attendances and admissions, causing almost all other admitting beds to be occupied at least once. The old bunk-beds joke had already been used more than once in paediatric nurse practitioner team huddles.

Several elective surgical cases were in the hospital but were yet to be taken to theatre pending the necessary magic tricks to create a vacant bed for them to be admitted to post-surgery. The word 'elective' is something of a misnomer, defined as being 'chosen by the patient rather than urgently necessary'. In the children's hospital this could refer to vital cardiac surgery or a life-saving kidney transplant, for example.

One such 'elective' was a child awaiting an ear, nose and throat (ENT) procedure on his airway. The decision to operate had been informed by a diagnostic sleep study. This study showed, in the words of the robust yet close-to-tears paediatric ENT surgeon, that he couldn't be sure that the child wouldn't die if he went home without the procedure. Through what can only be described as a leap of faith we collectively agreed that the procedure should be performed.

While the surgeon started work, several other senior nursing, medical and managerial staff got busy boxing, coxing and conjuring to somehow free up the paediatric intensive care bed that the boy would initially need post-surgery. The process essentially involves moving children around hospital beds like the most valuable jigsaw pieces imaginable while discussing, deliberating and negotiating with a multitude of clinical teams to ensure risk is absolutely minimised. In this instance, due to the indescribable commitment and ingenuity of staff and some genuine patience from the young boy's parents, the NHS gods smiled.

## Improvement needs time and space

The tendency of operational pressures of this kind to take precedence over work to improve how care is provided is a constant risk. It takes strong leadership and relationships between the NHS provider, commissioners, regulators and government to accept that teams must have time and space to review how they work. This means spending less time reporting on what they do and responding to the demands of trust leaders and the regulators in order to create more opportunities to improve. As the saying goes, it means working smarter not harder.

The manager's role in improving care will vary depending on experience, personality type, values and team dynamics. My approach is to develop strong, positive and optimistic relationships with my clinical teams that enable open communication and proactive planning. To facilitate this way of working, I work with different teams to establish their future visions and action plans to support implementation. My role is to ensure pragmatic steps are taken to help us towards our vision, championing Plan-Do-Study-Act (PDSA) principles and helping teams to focus on improving care delivery even in the face of intense operational pressures.

A tangible example is the establishment of a telephone advice line for GPs known as the Children's Assessment and Referral Service (CARS). The origins of the service can be found in a review of data showing that many patients were referred by GPs to an outpatient clinic, and were seen and discharged or seen and subsequently attended A&E. We decided to pilot a telephone hotline that GPs could call for advice with the patient in front of them. If appropriate, GPs could refer the patient to a general paediatric 'hot clinic' within 24 to 48 hours rather than the patient attending A&E or indeed deteriorating at home. CARS has proved to be a success, with positive feedback from GPs and support from commissioners.

We were able to set up CARS by borrowing a colleague to provide project management support and taking a financial risk within the directorate in which I work. The staff involved carried out the work for the pilot in their own time alongside their other responsibilities. As this example shows, improvements in care are possible but they rely on the discretionary effort of clinical teams and the managers who support them, and they have to compete for time and attention against the many other demands facing them.

If I were to sum up the job of being a hospital manager at the current time, it would be:

- work with clinical teams to develop the best possible clinical services and associated reputation within the resources available

- strive to develop a culture where saying 'yes' to patients/referring colleagues is the default

- develop plans to accommodate more patients through doing things differently, shifting care, adopting lean and other continuous improvement methodologies

- be delighted by the fantastic progress made

- be staggered that the rate of progress achieved today – which was significantly greater than the rate of progress yesterday or ever before – will be significantly short of the rate of progress required tomorrow

- return to the top of this list and do it all again…

## A Care Quality Commission perspective: Mike Richards

*Mike Richards is the Chief Inspector of Hospitals at the Care Quality Commission (CQC). He was National Cancer Director for 13 years before joining CQC in 2013 and was an oncologist and Professor of Palliative Medicine before that. He is passionately committed to improving the quality of care for patients across the country, with transparent assessment being a fundamental driver for change.*

Between September 2013 and March 2016 the CQC undertook comprehensive inspections of all 136 acute NHS trusts in England. These inspections used a new methodology that assesses and rates eight core services in each acute hospital on five high-level key questions.

- Is it safe?

- Is it effective?

- Is it caring?

- Is it responsive to patients' needs?

- Is it well led?

Each of these services/key questions is rated on a four-point scale (outstanding, good, requires improvement, inadequate). These individual ratings are then aggregated to give ratings for each core service and ultimately a rating for the trust as a whole.

This programme of inspections has provided us with a unique perspective on the quality of care being provided within the NHS. The depth and breadth of published information on quality of care in the NHS is probably unrivalled across the world. Our inspections have revealed wide variations in the quality of care being delivered to patients, both between hospitals and within hospitals. Perhaps unsurprisingly, we find the greatest number of concerns in emergency departments and in medical care. This is a reflection of the pressures that the NHS is facing with increasing emergency attendances and admissions, the rising numbers of frail or older patients with multiple morbidities and the difficulty with discharging patients when they are medically fit.

## Features of outstanding trusts

Five of the 136 acute trusts were rated as outstanding at their first comprehensive inspection and one has been given a rating of outstanding on re-inspection. These are:

- Frimley Health NHS Foundation Trust

- Salford Royal NHS Foundation Trust

- Western Sussex Hospitals NHS Foundation Trust

- Northumbria Healthcare NHS Foundation Trust

- The Newcastle Upon Tyne Hospitals NHS Foundation Trust

- University Hospitals Bristol NHS Foundation Trust.

In addition, five specialist NHS trusts, two mental health trusts and one ambulance trust have been rated as outstanding, representing around 6 per cent of all 238 NHS trusts. It is also important to note that trusts rated as good or requiring

improvement overall may have individual services that are rated as outstanding (Care Quality Commission 2017).

What features distinguish these outstanding trusts? Based on the findings from CQC inspections and in-depth conversations with leaders of almost all of these organisations, I have observed the following characteristics:

- A passion for high-quality, patient-centred care among the trust's leadership. This is observable not only in conversations in their offices but also when they are walking through the wards and corridors of their hospitals, talking to staff and patients.

- A clear strategic direction, based on a good understanding of the trust's strengths and weaknesses, and of the external environment.

- Good governance processes – knowing where problems are arising at the earliest opportunity and then dealing with them.

- Good engagement with and support for staff, listening and acting on issues that can be resolved. Management and staff being aligned on the central purpose of delivering the best possible care to patients.

- The ability to take tough decisions when needed.

- A focus on organisational development and quality improvement. These need to go hand-in-hand. The precise approach to quality improvement does not appear to be critical, as long as the trust has an agreed approach.

In several outstanding hospitals and mental health services in both the United Kingdom and the United States, the starting point for improvement was a 'burning platform'. This could be either an individual tragic case or a recognition of serious underlying problems, such as high mortality rates. The key point in these organisations that have gone on to be outstanding is that they have been open about their problems and determined to do better.

## Outstanding does not mean perfect

None of the outstanding trusts in England is perfect. Most importantly they would all openly acknowledge this. Indeed, CQC's ratings grids show this, with individual cells or core services on the grids being rated as requiring improvement, while the overall picture is one of good and outstanding ratings. This was the case when we inspected Western Sussex in December 2015: at that time 10 of 18 core services across three locations were rated as outstanding, 6 were rated as good and 2 were rated as requiring improvement.

The CQC provider handbooks (CQC 2016) describe the characteristics of outstanding and we assess trusts against these characteristics whenever an inspection team proposes a rating of outstanding. What we are looking for is something special that marks a service out from others – and that others could therefore learn from. However, we fully recognise that many NHS trusts have buildings and IT systems that are very far from ideal, and that make the working lives of clinical staff more onerous than they need to be.

The comments made by others in this series of papers about IT systems at Western Sussex therefore come as no surprise to me. I note that their comments relate both to IT systems within the trust and with cross-boundary communication with general practices and other hospitals. Both of these clearly need attention locally and nationally.

## Cross-boundary working

CQC's current statutory remit is to assess the quality and safety of individual provider organisations, whether these are hospitals, GP practices, care homes or other health and social care facilities. However, we fully recognise the importance to patients and to clinicians of cross-boundary working and communication. Chris Ham and Don Berwick highlight the deficiencies in these links at present in the Introduction to this report.

The assessment of cross-boundary or pathway working is one that CQC is keen to explore further. I believe we can do this by asking relevant questions of a range of key stakeholders and by incorporating these into our future assessments and ratings of hospitals. For example, we could ask local GPs how easy it is to get advice from specialists by phone or email and how rapidly they receive information after a patient is discharged. We could also ask referring hospitals to comment on how well they are served by specialist centres and vice versa.

I was interested that one of the cases mentioned by Chris Ham and Don Berwick related to the difficulty of getting information about a cancer patient who had been treated at another hospital. I believe that cancer services would be a very good model for the assessment of pathway or cross-boundary working. This is of particular importance when a patient is treated at one hospital but then presents as an emergency to another hospital. Immediate access to information can be vital.

### Conclusion

No hospital in England or the world is perfect, or ever will be. There will always be room for innovation and improvement. We do have some outstanding trusts and services but the fantastic care delivered to patients is often over-reliant on staff going beyond what can reasonably be expected of them. Patients and staff deserve better facilities and IT systems to assist them in delivering outstanding care.

## A patient safety director's perspective: Mike Durkin

*Mike Durkin is the NHS National Director of Patient Safety at NHS Improvement. He was previously the Medical Director of the South of England Strategic Health Authority having held executive medical director positions at strategic health authorities and at Gloucestershire Royal Hospital.*

When I read about the changes put in place at Western Sussex Hospitals NHS Foundation Trust, I felt an immediate association with its journey. It shines a light for many of us as we try to understand how to improve the care we offer while at the same time maintaining the delivery of effective care in an increasingly pressurised system. It also highlights the risks to patient safety even when staff are working to the best of their abilities.

Leaders at Western Sussex recognised the need to align the leadership and ward staff around the goals, methods and – I would add – values of their quality model, Patients First. This is a key principle put forward by Gary Kaplan at the Virginia Mason Medical Center but it is also a key principle shaping how the NHS already succeeds in delivering high-quality care most of the time. Our goal therefore is to learn how to do this every time a patient needs care and at every interface of a patient's transition along his or her journey.

Three things matter. First, we need to understand more about what is going wrong in the thousands of different pathways of care that are offered to our patients. Second, once we have some reliable data sources about what is happening, we need to put in place the capacity and capability to improve at every level of our system. Third, we need to get serious about tackling the underlying barriers to widespread safety improvement.

These barriers are not just the known avoidable harms such as falls, pressure ulcers, health care-associated infections and sepsis. They are also the insidious barriers that have often undone our own personal confidence and esteem as practitioners of health care: a lack of openness and candour, a fear of reporting a mistake, insufficient appropriate information, and often a lack of trust and respect among ourselves as executives, managers and frontline health care workers. If we are not working together with and for our patients, we are letting them and ourselves down when they need us most.

Avedis Donabedian was a wonderful educator and architect of quality improvement who taught us about the relationship of structure, process and outcome in health care. He reminds us that systems' awareness and systems' design are important for health professionals. But they are not enough: it is the ethical commitments of the individuals providing care that are essential to a system's success.

## A relevant model

The time and space to improve are precious and rare in the NHS and require extraordinary leadership at every level of care. One of the key elements is the ability to develop a model of quality that is relevant to everyone who delivers care. This applies wherever care is provided: in hospitals, general practices, urgent care centres, care homes and other settings.

We have had many opportunities to learn how to develop good health care quality. Examples include the work of the Institute of Medicine in *To err is human* (Kohn *et al* 2000) and *Crossing the quality chasm* (Institute of Medicine 2000); Sir Liam Donaldson as Chief Medical Officer describing the principles of good clinical governance in *An organisation with a memory* (Department of Health Expert Group 2000); and more recently from Ara Darzi's model in *High quality care for all* (Department of Health 2008). We are now at a time when we must build on these models and recognise the importance of two further elements to add to patient experience and safety, effectiveness and efficiency, and productivity and access.

These two further elements, namely the values of the individuals working within the system and the value that the quality model adds to organisation it serves, bring together a suite of fundamental principles enabling a return to good clinical governance principles. They should remain at the forefront of our relationship with our patients, our teams and our leaders. As the NHS becomes more and more pressurised through dealing with an increasing level of demand, it becomes more important for leaders of the system to support staff and patients at every stage of a patient's clinical journey.

Without true reliable and resilient systems of handover, we allow risk to escalate and avoidable harms to occur. We need to work hard to align the values of the board, the executive and operational managers with those of clinical staff and patients. Effective handover is just one vital element in the transformation that is required to create a truly effective team and system.

We should use all available tools. This means ensuring the transparency of our data sources by publishing and reporting our quality metrics; sharing data between and across all organisations along our patients' pathways; insisting that there is true candour when things go wrong; and recognising the balance of harm that can affect the staff involved in the incident as well as the patient and their family no matter how unintended.

## Commitment and compassion

I was reminded a few days ago of the allegory of the two wolves.

An old Cherokee is teaching his grandson about life. 'A fight is going on inside me,' he said to the boy. 'It is a terrible fight and it is between two wolves. One is evil – he is anger, envy, sorrow, regret, greed, arrogance, self pity, guilt, resentment, inferiority, lies, false pride, superiority and ego.' He continued: 'The other is good – he is joy, peace, love, hope, serenity, humility, kindness, benevolence, empathy, generosity, truth, compassion and faith. The same fight is going on inside you – and inside every other person too.' The grandson thought about it for a minute and then asked his grandfather, 'Which wolf will win?'

The old Cherokee simply replied, 'The one you feed'.

As Donabedian said, 'ultimately the secret of quality is love' (Mullan 2001). He believed as I do that it is the love of commitment and compassion that matters. A commitment to each other no matter what the circumstance, and compassion for each other, whether that be as a patient or a colleague.

So here are three final thoughts in reflecting on the path to support our staff and patients when they are at their most fragile and pressurised.

- Align the ethical values of all those involved in providing care, from board to ward, from the practice to the patient and from the care home assistant to the resident.

- Support with empathy and compassion all who work in health care, recognising the value that each person brings to the conversation with patients.

- Support leaders at every level who need to know that we as staff are always willing to go the extra mile if they are willing to repay our commitment.

The commitment of love that we show for our families, our patients, our teams and our hospitals and practices holds the key to delivering safe care to patients every time.

#  How could clinical care be improved?

## A quality improvement champion's perspective: Don Berwick

*Don Berwick was the founding chief executive of the Institute for Healthcare Improvement, US. He was the Administrator of the Centers for Medicare and Medicaid Services until December 2011. In 2013 he carried out a review of patient safety in the NHS on behalf of Prime Minister David Cameron. Don has authored or co-authored more than 160 scientific articles and six books.*

This project began rather accidentally. In 2015 I became an International Visiting Fellow at The King's Fund, with a specific focus on NHS England's new care models programme.

Around that time, unanticipated emails began arriving from a British physician, Gordon Caldwell, who was a stranger to me then but he issued a friendly challenge – in effect: 'Come and visit me on my hospital rounds some time, and get a real sense of what is happening at the coalface of care.'

Gordon was working at Worthing Hospital, part of the Western Sussex Hospitals NHS Foundation Trust, which had received high levels of recognition from the Care Quality Commission. I decided to take Gordon up on his challenge in June 2016. Our introduction to this report tells the story of my visit to Worthing and my experience on rounds with Gordon in more detail, along with a follow-up visit by my King's Fund colleague, Chris Ham.

In broad strokes, Chris and I saw an anomaly: on the one hand, we observed serious and costly problems at Gordon's 'coalface' – missing and inaccessible information, unreliable support processes, dysfunctional spaces for care and ever-present delays. On the other hand, we met a hospital management team committed to excellence, well tutored in modern approaches to improvement and celebrating many important innovations. In Marianne Griffiths it had a chief executive whose expertise in improvement and commitment to change could not have been more impressive.

How was this possible? How, in an award-winning hospital with a track record of innovation, results and enviable senior leadership teamwork, could there be at least one ward, on one afternoon, with doctors, patients and staff struggling to get even the basics of care right?

Three questions took shape for me that June day.

- Are the 'coalface' problems we observed widespread in the NHS, or were that day and that place exceptions?

- Why were the problems there?

- What could be done about them?

These became the organising questions for The King's Fund appreciative inquiry represented in these pages.

## Go to the gemba

As a student of quality and improvement for four decades, I was in some ways already familiar with such a story and its apparent paradox. One of the most useful framings for me came from Japanese quality scholars who had been my tutors in years past, most importantly Professor Noriaki Kano, from the University of Tokyo. Though little known in the United States or the United Kingdom, Professor Kano is a towering figure in the global community of teachers and researchers on quality management.

His most often-cited contributions concern systematic approaches to understanding and designing for customers' need, both overt and latent. He has also mentored practitioners for decades on how to achieve rapid, scientifically grounded process improvement. In this, he is relentless about the need for leaders to 'go to the gemba', gemba being a Japanese term for 'the shop floor' or 'the place where the work is done'.

Experts like Kano believe that few errors in management are more consequential – or more common – than the loss of touch between the executive suite and the settings of day-to-day work. When leaders and workers fall out of touch with each other, misunderstandings arise, investments get misaligned, and both parties lose access to the real-world data that they need in order to learn, test changes and make progress. Scientifically grounded improvement depends on widespread tests of change, constant inquiry and observation, and continual adaptation to ever-changing circumstances at the local level. Going to the gemba is essential for such learning and iteration.

The dissonance between the evident skill and achievements of Worthing's leadership team and the problems I saw on rounds with Gordon raised some questions. Is there a gap in understanding between the leaders and the gemba at Worthing? And, if so, how can it be remedied? And, if misunderstanding is not the culprit, what is?

In my three decades of experience in the pursuit of continual improvement in health care, I have come to believe that gaps in understanding between senior executive teams and the world of daily work are common, despite the skill and commitment of both. Senior leaders live in a world that uses the language of finance and strategy, keeping their eyes on external threats and opportunities, trying to perceive and react to big-picture tectonics and patterns. Those in daily work use the language of care, keep their eyes on local operations, and feel that finance and strategy are beyond their control and, frankly, less interesting than the tasks immediately before them.

I have seen chief executives of billion-dollar hospitals stop at the entry to clinical areas as if they were travellers at a border without a passport. And I have seen frontline doctors and nurses who have never set foot in the executive offices of the organisations that employ them, but who nonetheless criticise those executives, whose work they do not understand.

The consequence of these different worldviews is that the priorities and circumstances of each party – executive and frontline – are, at best, incompletely understood by and, at worst, unknown to the other. Executives feel frustrated that clinicians don't seem to understand the stresses on the corporation; and clinicians and other staff mutter that the executives ought to 'come down here and see what it's really like!'.

### Closing the divide

The best organisations try actively to close that divide. At the heart of many improvement methodologies – such as six-sigma, lean production, 'kaizen' and 'quality circles' – lie mechanisms to bring frontline knowledge and executive skills closer to each other. At the Virginia Mason Medical Center, for example, which is devoted to mastery of its version of the Toyota Production System, every day you will find executive teams huddling on local units with frontline staff in front of storyboards and charts displaying the real conditions of local care and outcomes.

Executive walk-arounds are happily becoming more and more common. Quality improvement teams comprise diagonal slices of an organisation's hierarchy. This is how the military approaches 'after action reviews', in which everyone from general to private leaves rank at the door and engages in searching conversations about what happened, why, and what could have been better.

Such 'sensitivity to operations' is one of the key aspects of Professor Karl Weick's framework for 'high-reliability organisations'. 'If a wrench is left on the flight deck of an aircraft carrier,' Weick writes, 'the Admiral will know' (Weick and Sutcliffe 2001).

The fact that distance could develop between Gordon's daily world and the extraordinary leadership team at Worthing is no comment on the competence of either. Indeed, several of the essays in this series testify to the extraordinary skill of Worthing's leaders in centring their strategy on the continual improvement of care. Rather, it is a comment on how truly difficult it is to bridge between the executive suite and the gemba.

In the specific case of Worthing, the 'index case' for this appreciative inquiry, it would be very hard to believe that Gordon's world is not, in fact, well understood by a leadership team fully schooled in world-class quality improvement methods. Additional factors must be in play, and, as the essays in this report testify, serious resource constraints in the context of rising demand may offer at least some explanation.

The task of improving daily work is always demanding, but especially so when resources are squeezed. We heard time and again that the NHS in England is now under nearly unbearable financial constraints, whose effects are worsened by both rising demographic demands and by the persistence of flawed processes of care.

Under such pressure, both staff and leaders have trouble merely surviving their day-to-day work, let alone innovating. Paradoxically, just when process improvement, wise standardisation, innovation, a focus on safety and buoying workforce morale become most important, they actually come under most jeopardy.

How can the NHS avoid this vicious cycle? And, in service of continually better and more efficient care, how can leaders and the front line come together most effectively to protect their shared mission?

The first step, we believe, needs to be serious, honest and respectful inquiry. For starters, what are the extent and nature of process failures in acute care in NHS trusts, of the types we saw with Dr Caldwell? Why are they there? And what can be done to fix them, by whom?

As outlined in the Introduction, these essays, and the roundtable discussions they capture, form a first contribution to that inquiry. Unsurprisingly, neither the answers nor the suggestions that came forth proved uniform or simple. But the emerging picture is pregnant with possibilities for improved care.

And that, in many ways, is the main point that we hope will emerge from these writings. That, as in any complex, interdependent system, nurturing understanding of the real world of daily work – the gemba – in the NHS is a never-ending task, well worth the time and investment of leaders at all levels.

## A quality improver's perspective: Bob Klaber

*Bob Klaber is a consultant general paediatrician at Imperial College Healthcare NHS Trust. He has a strong interest in learning, improvement and leadership development and through his associate medical director role is now leading work to create a culture of improvement across the organisation. Bob also co-leads the Connecting Care for Children integrated child health programme.*

I feel extremely privileged to work both as a general paediatrician and in a senior trust-wide leadership role, which together give me some interesting perspectives on this gap between senior leadership and frontline staff. My work as a paediatrician involves 'attending weeks' and on-calls on our inpatient ward, outpatient clinics, leading multidisciplinary teams in primary care and support for colleagues seeing children and young people in the Emergency Department. My trust-wide role is leading a small quality improvement team with the aim of creating a culture of continuous improvement across the organisation.

We began developing our quality improvement programme at the trust in 2015, building both on our quality strategy and, equally importantly, on a powerful staff-led engagement project that revisited what staff and patients felt were the most important values and behaviours for our organisation. The messages from this work were clear: first, that we needed to put emphasis on values such as being kind and collaborative, and second, that this had to be about real behaviours, not just a set of words at the bottom of a letterhead. The most important measure of this would be how the organisation felt to work in, or to be a patient in, and so a focus on how we all behave, and the relationships and connections we build, would be the ultimate determinant of that.

Quality improvement can sometimes come across as predominantly a technical science, but it was clear to us that our main focus should be on engagement: supporting, facilitating and encouraging our staff, patients and families to identify and make improvements themselves. In order to achieve our 10- to 20-year aim of creating an organisational culture of continuous improvement we feel there are four areas, or drivers, where we need to focus our efforts, and my guess is that these would apply in most other health care organisations.

- Engage with staff to ensure everyone feels empowered and energised to see improving care as a key part of their role.

- Build improvement capability through a programme of quality improvement education that enables staff to lead, champion and coach improvement activities within their teams.

- Support teams to deliver focused improvement projects and programmes that are co-designed with patients, service-users and the public.

- Embed consistent and rigorous improvement methods in all our work across the organisation.

We are working hard on each of these drivers and, 18 months in, are making good progress. Reflecting on some of the successes, the improvement work that has been the most impactful has been where leaders and teams from across the organisation have come together to work collaboratively on team-initiated projects that start at the gemba but align with organisational strategic priorities.

Examples include collaborative work to improve the uptake and quality of clinical coding and service transformation work that has originated from co-design events involving patients and the public. Our 'QI sprints', based loosely on the design principles of a hackathon [a design event in which computer programmers and others collaborate intensively on software projects], have been a great way to bring together service-users, health care and other professionals to design and plan improvements. Within this approach is a consistency and equality of language that is an enabler for close teamworking and also leads to a positive sense of achievement and purpose in work through the gains made.

## Halting adversarial behaviours

One theme that has come to the fore in all this work has been the importance of finding the right 'tone' in everything we do. What I mean by tone is the way we speak to each other, how hard we listen, the approach we use to challenge and the efforts we put in to give encouragement and support. Although there are many rewards, health care is an extraordinarily tough environment in which to work, and yet too often it is made harder by the way we behave to each other.

It seems that this is particularly problematic across perceived boundaries, be they organisational or professional. Whether it is doctor–manager, commissioner–provider, consultant–GP, regulator–trust, senior–junior, it seems to increase the chances of people rubbishing each other and taking an adversarial approach to communication. I am totally clear that we need to be rigorous and robust in the standards we set and in our expectations around quality, safety and experience and, where performance is falling short, this needs to be addressed. However, if we are really to transform health care into a more person-centred, efficient and compassionate delivery model we all need to play our part in putting a halt to these adversarial behaviours.

The aggressive and combative tone that one sees across different areas of health care needs to be systematically highlighted and pushed back on, wherever it is originating. The effect of these behaviours, that in reality are a form of bullying, is almost always counter-productive and can sometimes be devastating. The implications are magnified when they are coming from someone in a senior position. This is not about avoiding difficult conversations: on the contrary, it is about having them in a civilised, thoughtful and constructive way that builds trust and relationships and is much more likely to deliver the outcomes our patients deserve.

As well as standing up to situations where these destructive behaviours are playing out, we all have a role in setting the right tone and culture in the microsystems within which we are working. Examples of this include consistent use of first names across traditional team hierarchies and senior leaders proactively making themselves visible and accessible to all staff. These small but important behaviours are crucial as they create the psychological safety for more junior staff to test ideas and make improvements.

My final reflection relates to my understanding that staff are more likely to succeed, stay and flourish within our NHS if they are learning, developing, feeling properly supported and have a clear sense of purpose in their work. Where the gap between senior leaders and the staff who are delivering care is wide, one can see that people are less likely to have clarity about how their role fits into the wider system, may feel unsupported and often have little sense of continuous learning. Each of us, wherever we find ourselves within the health care system, can positively influence this in our own small way. We can all do things to step across the hierarchical gaps that surround us; we can listen – listen really hard – and then move forward as a team with the benefit of the new perspectives we have gained.

## A medical director and chief executive's perspective: David Evans

*David Evans has been Chief Executive at Northumbria NHS Foundation Trust since November 2015. Previous to holding this post he was Medical Director for 12 years and Clinical Director for 8 years. David has been involved in developing and leading major clinical services changes, clinical governance and safety. Innovation and integration based on improving outcomes has been key to his working. He has been a consultant obstetrician and gynaecologist for 28 years.*

Northumbria NHS Foundation Trust faces some unusual challenges compared to many NHS providers. We serve 503,000 people spread over 2,500 square miles. Around 85 per cent of our population live in urban areas, leaving 15 per cent spread across one of the most remote parts of England. We provide not only acute care but also community nursing and therapy services. Adult social care is provided by the foundation trust under a Section 75 agreement with Northumberland County Council.

We support nine inpatient sites, a new-build specialist emergency care hospital that united the emergency streams for our three district general hospitals and which opened in June 2015, and five community hospitals delivering care to our rural population. We perform surgery on six sites and provide outpatient services from 13 sites. A system that supports such a diverse service has required tailored and specific solutions.

A key development has been to establish the role of chief clinical information officer, a post shared by a hospital consultant and a general practitioner. This post provides better understanding of whole-system working and created strategies and developments that deliver improved access to information for all parts of the service. It also overcame what had been traditional blocks to information exchange. This was chiefly due to a lack of understanding about how information governance rules can support the safe and secure sharing of patient data rather than stop that process.

### Inpatient services

In inpatient services we used an Oracle integration engine to unite information from our existing systems to create a single view of patients' records. This was the nearest we could get to an electronic patient record within the limitations of these systems. It means that on a single screen we can access the following information from any of our inpatient sites:

- patient demographics in a standard format

- test requests and results including live alerts and 'pending result' flagging

- a digital dictation archive of all letters/summaries

- an image archive and text reports

- worksheets including current messaging, eg, consultation requests.

We will soon add electronic prescribing after a lengthy search to find a system able to meet our needs.

In 2017 we will be implementing 'Nerve Centre'. This is a central monitoring system for all inpatients with automation of bedside recording and a central alert and advice function. Nerve Centre will also provide a trust-wide tracking system that will greatly aid bed management and patient movements.

We have centralised all our intensive care beds onto our new site. To support staff at our other hospitals we have replaced the former critical care outreach service with a system we call '7777'. At any time when advice and support are needed, or if a patient's early warning score reaches a critical level, a phone conversation takes place using an iPad via a secure web-based portal. This enables advice to be sought from an intensivist who can see the patient and discuss treatment options with the attending specialist.

## Community services

Linking diverse community services across a wide area has been a great challenge. Thanks to the efforts of many people, we have recently introduced the medical interoperability gateway using one of the main IT systems used by GPs. The gateway gives live access to appropriate patient information held by GPs to district nurses, therapists, pharmacists, social workers and clinicians in acute hospitals. It has supported agile working by staff in the community.

This breakthrough has transformed the safety and efficiency of our service. We have seen huge improvements in child protection and the management of vulnerable adults, in medicines management and reconciliation, and in multi-agency working. District nurses claim that they are able to see four extra patients each day because they no longer need to return to base to gather information. Although coverage is not perfect across our rural areas, even our most far-flung staff have hot-spots that they can identify to link up rather than having to make a 30-mile round trip to base.

The next step, building on '7777', is to use our tablet-based cameras to enable hospital-based specialists to offer advice in a patient's own home, in care or nursing homes and at GP surgeries. Based on what we have seen from other national initiatives such as those being used in Airedale, this could have a major impact on the need for patients to attend hospitals. We are also keen to explore how we could extend access to paramedics and first responders.

For some time we have run a 'virtual' fracture clinic at Berwick-upon-Tweed, situated more than 60 miles from an acute site. A consultant orthopaedic surgeon on one of our acute sites can view x-rays taken in the community hospital and can hold a face-to-face exchange via our web portal. For the vast majority of patients, appropriate care can be delivered locally and only those who need surgery have to travel. The potential is enormous for using this technology for a wide range of treatment reviews where tests can be taken locally and reviewed remotely.

## Lessons learnt

The gains we have made have been achieved by evolution and small-scale incremental developments rather than by a major systems change. Key to all of them has been the ownership by frontline clinical teams. We have made the products fit for the service rather than having to shoehorn clinical pathways into ready-made systems.

The blurring of traditional boundaries between primary and secondary care has been a key principle. Having joint leadership of these changes from both sectors has also been a major benefit. The shared understanding that this has brought to process redesign has allowed rapid change without the need for negotiation and revision.

Our systems will continue to evolve. In particular, agile working for community staff and the possibility of increasing the use of virtual clinics are important developments for a trust that serves a large rural population.

## A nurse's perspective: Clare Carter-Jones

*Clare Carter-Jones is cardiology matron at the Royal Free London NHS Foundation Trust. After nine years' A&E experience, Clare moved to senior nursing positions in acute medicine, respiratory and cardiology. She gained a Masters in clinical research*

*from St George's, University of London in 2011. Clare is a visible clinical leader and a passionate advocate for quality improvement.*

As a matron in a large London NHS trust, I lead two clinical areas and manage a team of around 75 nurses including two clinical nurse specialist teams. An important and rewarding part of my role has been leading quality improvement work and developing the talent within my team.

As in Worthing, the pressure that clinical staff here are under is enormous. Every day, we have operational pressures to manage with disjointed systems, compounded by poor communication. This is not only between teams – as a senior nurse I witness poor communication and handover processes from shift to shift and day to day. With so many people involved in any one patient's care, maintaining consistent information from staff member to staff member is incredibly challenging.

In recent times, we had a patient who was cared for on my ward for a period of many weeks. From a clinical perspective, he received expert consultant-led care in a tertiary centre; he had three specialist teams, expert in their fields, giving valuable input into his care; and he was nursed in a level two hospital bed with specialist trained nurses. His prognosis was very poor on admission and, despite being given every chance, he sadly died.

When I sat down and listened to the experience of his daughters, they described an exceptionally different hospital stay to that seen from the clinical perspective. In an articulate and dignified way, they told me they felt that we had been dishonest with them throughout their journey. They felt that each time a different team arrived to review their father, the doctor asked either them or their father what the plan was from the other teams; they appeared neither to read the notes nor communicate with the teams. The different messages, the friendly questions, the mistakes in history-taking and the lack of clarity with the clinical plan meant that the family never felt that they could entirely trust us to keep him safe.

They observed him being taken for procedures and tests with no nursing communication between the two teams about important aspects like fluid balance, cognition or comfort. Nurses and doctors gave different information and messages about progress, and when the family asked very intelligent questions of a registrar about ceilings of care, they were not answered. His death then came as a surprise, his resuscitation status only discussed in the last hours of his life and his family was not present for his last moments.

## Tests of change

No matter how incredibly capable and gifted we are as individuals, as a team and as teams working with teams, we can get this very wrong – as this one experience clearly illustrates. We are not supported by systems or cultures that encourage good communication. Of course, this is just one example, and in spite of all of this I have cards and letters that testify to the great care we provide most of the time. But this experience happened on my watch, with my team, and in my hospital. Their experience lives with me every day. I am motivated by the guilt and shame of one patient's experience to improve the care for all.

I'm incredibly lucky to work with a motivated team who are champions for the quality improvement work being done in our area. We have thought at length about what we do and why. We have asked each other about what matters to us and we have reflected on the data available to us about patient experience.

I talk a lot to my team about 'holding your nerve' through tests of change – but the phrase used by Marianne Griffiths, the Western Sussex chief executive, about 'strategic patience' is probably a more eloquent way of describing the agonising process of leading change and supporting teams through it. We have made no huge breakthroughs, but we have spent a lot of time on marginal gains – all of which I'm proud of my team for pushing through and having the confidence to test. These have included the following.

- We abolished 'nursing notes' and now write in the medical notes along with all other multidisciplinary team (MDT) members.

- We continue to test different ways to hand over as a nursing team and what that handover should entail – my dream would be to have doctors, nurses and therapists all starting the day together with one handover rather than staggered repeated meetings for different professions.

- However, we now have one handover database (therapists, nurses, doctors) instead of three, and even have found a way of having test results automatically fed through to this database to save time for the doctors in the morning.

- We are testing a new consultant-led MDT, which pulls together the relevant teams once a week, supported by our palliative care team and patient-at-risk and resuscitation team who can challenge/support difficult decision-making and enable clarity on ceilings of care.

- Morning board rounds are being restructured to highlight nursing concerns about patients and to allow the chance for anyone complex to be brought to the new weekly MDT.

London is not unusual in facing challenges with vacancies in the nursing workforce, which inevitably results in high turnover of staff. As a clinical leader I see my role as pivotal in recruiting staff on their values and capability, and developing their confidence along the way.

This means that they learn how to expand their sphere of influence beyond their peers, their profession and their clinical areas – to experience how to gain strategic influence, which is essential to all quality improvement. Sadly, we don't always grow doctors and nurses who have insight into what compassionate and effective leadership looks like and I see this as our greatest opportunity for improvement.

Senior nurses need to develop talent and not be scared to support staff to try small tests of change. Every complaint, every incident report, every compliment is our opportunity to reflect on how we work and gain insight into what has become normalised and where we have potential focus for improvement.

## A physician's perspective: Matthew Lewis

*Matthew Lewis is a consultant in general medicine and gastroenterology at Sandwell and West Birmingham Hospitals NHS Trust. He is also a Visiting Fellow at The King's Fund, where he draws on his experience of full-time clinical work and more than a decade in clinical management, included working as group director for medicine and emergency care until 2016.*

The care of patients in hospital demands a strong doctor–patient relationship but the role of the wider multidisciplinary team (MDT) is often equally, if not more, important. While a joint publication by the Royal College of Physicians and the Royal College of Nursing (2012) described ward rounds as 'a key component of daily hospital activity', I would suggest that the addition of board rounds creates an even stronger platform for acute inpatient care.

At a time when many patients on acute medical wards are frail or older people, the input of the wider professional body is key to assessing, treating and discharging patients. Ideally, a ward round would bring together the consultant, junior doctors, senior nurse, pharmacist, therapists (occupational, physio-, speech and language) – and even the social worker – for several hours each week. In practice, this is difficult to achieve as most wards are not staffed to this level; also, such a sustained period of co-ordinated activity would mean that staff would be tied to the ward round when they could be seeing patients independently.

Board rounds are scheduled, daily discussions of patient care that include as many members of the MDT as possible – consultants, junior doctors, nurses, physiotherapists or occupational therapists are essential; pharmacists and social workers are desirable. As the RCP/RCN report pointed out, board rounds can be used to share information from relatives, prioritise tasks, delegate responsibilities and maximise the effectiveness of time spent with the patient. Each patient can be discussed in under a minute – including presenting complaint, diagnosis, management plan and expected discharge date – so most wards can complete this in 20 to 30 minutes.

After the board round, selected patients (starting with those who are sick or unstable, followed by potential discharges) are reviewed by the relevant professional team(s), which allows investigations or treatments to be initiated earlier in the day and offers more chance for discharges to take place before dark. The board round discussion determines 'an integrated management plan with estimated discharge date and physiological and functional criteria for discharge', as described in the clinical standards for seven-day services (NHS Improving Quality 2016). Subsequently, the medical team can review the remaining patients on the ward as normal.

Fundamentally, the board round needs to have all the right clinical staff together, so the team must decide on timing and commit to being punctual – anything less is disrespectful to fellow professionals. Location is important because board rounds should not take place on the open ward where there are distractions from phones, food trolleys and other staff; confidentiality is a pre-requisite. Like any meeting, it needs to be well-chaired, so that the information can be shared succinctly and all the decisions made without unnecessary dialogue; in-depth clinical debates should take place after the board round as these usually involve only a single professional team. Lastly, each person needs to leave the board round with a clear idea of their tasks.

## Making board rounds successful

What makes a highly successful board round? Staff who know (and respect) each other can provide a valuable challenge – how will that scan change our management, why don't we try to help him to walk, what is to be gained from keeping this patient in hospital another couple of days, and so on. A trusting team will accept (even welcome) challenges from colleagues and will hold each other to account on a daily basis. The ability to verify the information that is recorded helps to ensure that errors are not being passed on inadvertently. Our board rounds all take place with a large screen in view of the whole MDT so that anyone can pick up mistakes and correct them immediately (the screen shows extensive information including diagnosis, social situation, therapy reviews and resuscitation status).

Information generated by the board round needs to be accessible promptly from any point in the hospital. So all medicine board rounds at Sandwell and West Birmingham Hospitals, apart from the acute medical units, are completed by 9.30am. Currently, our software package can be accessed from any trust computer by the clinical teams (to aid patient care) and by the operational managers (to assist with bed capacity planning).

Consultant job plans have been adjusted to take account of these changed working arrangements. We still have longer ward rounds as well – where patients can be assessed in detail and relatives kept abreast of developments – but board rounds take place each day and consultants are expected to attend at least four days a week (out of five). On the days when a full ward round is not scheduled by the consultant, there is short interval to review selected patients prior to starting other activity, as clinics or procedures lists can be delayed until 10.00am.

## Best practice and improvements

To make sure that we were sharing best practice (and offering critical guidance), we carried out a peer review process in September 2015. One person from each ward (consultant, junior, nurse or therapist) attended another ward and gave feedback according to our defined criteria; two weeks later, a further visit was set up to check that the changes had been implemented.

The main themes that came out of this were that discharge planning needed to start sooner in the admission, tasks had to be assigned clearly to specified individuals, potential weekend discharges should be planned more carefully, discussions should include all MDT members (not just doctors) and that poor timekeeping by any participant either prevented full discussion of all the patients, or made everyone else run late. In Tayside, similar issues were addressed with good results through the use of video-enhanced reflective practice (Hellier *et al* 2015). Subsequently, colleagues have commented that board rounds have helped teams to get to know each other, understand one another's roles and work more collaboratively.

What could we do better? One aim should be to harmonise handover processes so that a single electronic database is used for all staff to share information between different professional teams. Like many trusts, we are moving towards a full electronic patient record and this offers us the chance to standardise the transfer of patient data and minimise repetition.

Traditional ward rounds will continue to be an element of good patient care but the development of board rounds will encourage timely, informative, multidisciplinary decisions that can be shared electronically with the operational management team.

## A geriatrician's perspective: Tom Downes

*Tom Downes is a consultant geriatrician at Sheffield Teaching Hospitals. He gained an MBA from Nottingham University Business School and subsequently a Masters in public health at Harvard. He undertook a Health Foundation Quality Improvement Fellowship at the Institute for Healthcare Improvement and on his return to Sheffield developed the role of clinical lead for quality improvement.*

Two years ago, I visited a Toyota factory and the strongest memory I had was of talking to a man whose job it was to fit seals to car door windows. He recalled how he had noticed that ensuring the seal was fitted tightly on both sides caused him to awkwardly crane round the door. He had the idea of fitting a mirror so that he could simultaneously see both sides of the seal as he fitted it, thereby removing the awkwardness and increasing efficiency. He worked in a culture in which reporting issues was positive and he was enabled to test his idea to discover an improvement. When the idea had been successfully implemented, it was rapidly spread across the organisation.

In health care, we need to be cautious when translating from other industries. My organisation has been developing the principles of 'see, solve, share and lead'. We train staff in the knowledge of improvement science and the skills of team coaching. Stable, enabling leadership has created the conditions for staff and patients to apply these skills to discover wide-ranging improvement, including new acute assessment processes, innovative discharge pathways and new models of long-term condition care.

We started on our journey of building quality improvement capability six years ago with a very small improvement team – initially just two improvement coaches testing the concept of team coaching combined with improvement science. As microsystem teams started to demonstrate improved outcomes and efficiency gains, the demand for coaching outstripped supply. We started the Sheffield Microsystem Coaching Academy in 2012 and are currently training our eighth cohort of microsystem improvement coaches.

Over the same six years we have been developing a translation of the Toyota 'oobeya' – the room from which Toyota prototypes, designs and launches new car model lines. Oobeya roughly translates to 'big room'. We set up our first Big Room to coach improvement across geriatric and community care. The first two 'products' launched from this weekly meeting were an acute frailty assessment unit and the flipped discharge concept of 'discharge to assess'. Implementation of these reduced geriatric medicine's bed occupancy by 30 per cent.

The second Big Room in Sheffield coached respiratory medicine staff, facilitating them to improve their service. They achieved significant reductions in both length of stay and mortality. A key factor in the success of this approach to improvement is ownership by the staff. The improvement coaches help the staff to improve their own work, focusing on what is important to them and their patients.

Combining our knowledge from training microsystem coaches with learning from two successful Big Rooms, we have developed a one-year action learning course for training pairs of staff (a manager and a clinician) to set up a Big Room and co-coach improvement across a condition-based pathway. There are now eleven Big Rooms in Sheffield and The Health Foundation is supporting us to replicate the model as a social franchise setting up Flow Coaching Academies. The second Flow Coaching Academy has started in Bath and within one year there will be five, with a further three each year.

The introduction to this report asks where responsibility should lie for mitigating and overcoming the difficulties. Potentially the answer is simple: it is 'high velocity learning by everyone, about everything, all of the time' (Spear 2017). In Sheffield, we are making progress towards this vision. We are getting better at providing the right conditions, for successful improvement work, through a combination of:

- leadership development

- helping teams share their success to increase confidence to free up people's time

- nurturing a network to provide peer support.

Together these conditions provide a platform of opportunity for staff to learn and engage with improvement. We have seen that the conditions for successful improvement work are complex and we continue to innovate to overcome the barriers – it is much more than simply training coaches. We have started to see the signs of cultural change and were encouraged last year when our CQC report noted 'a culture of innovation and improvement was evident throughout all levels of the organisation'.

While maintaining the focus on helping staff in our own organisation to improve their work, we are expanding our horizons. We already work collaboratively to develop improvement capability with our city's paediatric hospital, mental health trust and, increasingly, primary care. Much of our pathway improvement work naturally crosses organisational boundaries and our collaborative approach builds relationships and trust. Looking forward, we are aiming to learn how to accelerate and sustain our internal work while also forging an expanding external network of coaching academies to learn together.

## A clinical researcher's perspective: Sam Pannick

*Sam Pannick is a specialist registrar in gastroenterology and internal medicine at West Hertfordshire Hospitals NHS Trust. Sam studied pre-clinical medicine at the University of Cambridge and then graduated with distinction from the Royal Free and University College Medical School. He is a member of the Royal College of Physicians and holds a PhD from Imperial College London on the quality of medical ward care.*

Every ward has its own routine: different board rounds, different ward round styles, different multidisciplinary meetings. As a trainee physician, I wondered why the organisation of ward care was so arbitrary. After all, the medical ward is the fundamental care delivery unit for most hospitalised patients. It's a place of treatment, where patients receive therapy; a temporary home, where they take meals and receive their visitors; and – for many medical patients – a resting place, where they are comforted in their final days. These basic premises haven't changed since Florence Nightingale first highlighted the benefits of good ward design. Yet providing high-quality care in this setting still feels like an uphill struggle.

Nightingale herself focused on physical characteristics of the hospital environment: ventilation, light and hygiene. Modern researchers have now gone further, looking at ward processes and interdisciplinary care teams – as well as the bricks and mortar. Their work certainly bears out the difficulties we face on our wards: reliably delivering care in the NHS is immensely challenging, as our operational systems do not support it (Burnett *et al* 2012). Nurses spend 9 per cent of their time just working around 'routine' problems with the information and materials they depend on (Tucker 2004).

Still, with an explosion of academic articles about health care safety and quality in the past 15 years, I thought it would be relatively straightforward to identify the interventions that make ward care better. Instead, I've found two main challenges in my PhD on ward care.

- What medical wards do is varied, complex and difficult to articulate.

  High-quality ward care is easy to visualise, but much more difficult to define and measure. Medical wards treat a hugely diverse range of patients, and there isn't a consensus about the measurements that reflect good ward care in the United Kingdom. Studies of interdisciplinary interventions on medical wards use a variety of outcomes, from length of stay to readmissions and mortality, measured at various times all the way up to one year post-discharge (Pannick *et al* 2015). With so little agreement on the goals of ward care, or when to measure them, it's difficult to assess whether any intervention truly has its desired impact.

- There is little high-quality evidence for effective ward-level interventions.

  Ward-level interventions target five elements of care: team composition; interdisciplinary collaboration; care standardisation; early treatment of the deteriorating patient; and local safety climate (Pannick *et al* 2014). These are intuitively important – but there's surprisingly little evidence about how to change them for the better. There haven't been many rigorous trials of interdisciplinary ward interventions, particularly in the United Kingdom. Still, in the real world, tools like checklists have been widely adopted – mostly based on evidence from other clinical areas, like intensive care and operating theatres. But we've often introduced these tools onto the ward without a good understanding of how they might work best, or how to implement them. As a result, when we do test them, they can fail to live up to our expectations.

## Existing evidence

What have I learnt from the existing evidence on ward care? First, we need to be clearer on how we are judging ward quality. We should define the structures (inputs), processes (how we do things) and outcomes (including patient experience) that represent high-quality ward care in the United Kingdom. This formal approach would underpin a wider conversation about the many factors that influence ward care, from upstream supply chains to ward-level leadership. Without this clarity, we're putting the cart before the horse, introducing changes without really knowing what we're hoping to improve.

Second, our chosen quality metrics will improve only when our operational structures improve. Our focus to date on teamwork and collaboration has been laudable, but improvement does not rest on teamwork alone. For ward staff to fulfil their potential, teams must be empowered by work systems that make sense, not predispose them to error; by adequate staffing, not skeleton staffing; by smart equipment that nudges, not overwhelms; and by learning communities that build better practice.

We lionise frontline staff for their ability to get things done in a failing system; it is now time to address those failings. A continuous focus on the operational aspects of care delivery may be the only truly sustainable route to improvement (Bohmer 2016). This should encompass both the foundational structures of care (like supply chains, environment and information systems) as well as the interdisciplinary structures that organise care delivery each day.

Third, interdisciplinary ward interventions rarely work without sustained organisational backing. We need to be realistic about the resources and focus needed to change ward care. Complex interventions make a real impact when multiple factors come together: national pressure for change, financial incentives that reward implementation, and local investment and leadership. Ward care needs to be prioritised as an organisational objective, recognising that many of the challenges faced by ward teams arise in other departments and need managerial resolution. Staff-led change efforts can be embedded and sustained only with the help of managers who are incentivised to see quality improvement as a key component of their role (Pannick *et al* 2016a). This is a long game.

I don't think that improved ward care will come about entirely through off-the-shelf intervention packages. Wards are too complex for that. But the learning from previous successes and failures can be shared, and adapted, and implemented sensitively, to suit each new context (Dixon-Woods and Martin 2016). There are no magic bullets, but a movement for better ward care will hinge on having the right organisational and team structures, fostering reliable processes and more effective teamwork. We need to be much harder on our systems: this will help us be far, far kinder to our people.

## A Royal College of Physicians' perspective: Mark Temple

*Mark is a consultant physician and nephrologist, Heart of England Foundation Trust, Birmingham, where he led innovation of acute medical services as clinical director and associate medical director. Mark chaired the hospital pathways workstream of the Future Hospital Commission and was appointed Future Hospital Officer in 2014.*

For clinical staff on a good day the job is immensely rewarding. However, there is almost universal experience of dark days with staff unable to deliver the care they would like, striving to maintain basic standards of safe, effective care. When this happens day after day, in tandem with feeling unsupported, the personal cost can be considerable leading to demoralisation and burn-out.

Clinical pressures are such that finding a 'work around' is endemic with, for example, no time to report equipment failures immediately, compounded by little priority given to repair once reporting occurs. The malfunctioning laptop means the junior doctor has to leave the ward round to mine information on a desktop, missing the senior review of that patient.

In such a financially constrained environment the government, more than ever, needs to partner health care leaders to find and deliver new models of care. Supportive leadership is crucial. Sadly, recent messages have been more about blaming rather than valuing staff, talking up transformation and talking down the stark realities of the pressures on acute care in the NHS.

The unprecedented pressures on the NHS are well known. *Hospitals on the edge?* (Royal College of Physicians 2012) ascribed these to: changing patient needs (ageing population), increasing demand, fractured care, out-of-hours care breakdown and workforce crisis. *Underfunded, underdoctored, overstretched* (Royal College of Physicians 2016d) included the pressures of rising drug costs and cuts to the funding of social care and disease prevention. *Future Hospital: caring for medical patients* (Future Hospital Commission 2013) moved the national debate from diagnosing the NHS's ailments to prescribing treatment. The report described a model for the organisation of acute services, underpinned by a set of principles based on the needs of patients.

## Future Hospital Programme

The Royal College of Physicians (RCP) committed to testing the recommendations of the Future Hospital Commission's report through the Future Hospital Programme, and it launched the *Future Hospital Journal*. The core of the Future Hospital Programme is joint working with eight development sites in England and Wales, implementing recommendations relating to the care of older people with frailty and the delivery of new models of integrated care. The focus is on co-production with patients, using quality improvement methodology.

The programme sets out to create a collaborative community sharing the results of patient-centred, clinician-led incremental change. Models range from the Worthing emergency floor evaluating early specialist assessment of older people with frailty (including those on surgical pathways), to delivering telemedicine outpatient consultations in rural north Wales, and enhancing self-care and GP-led care of paediatric patients with severe allergies in north-west England. All the sites are 'real world' collaborations, with hard-pressed acute trust and community partners introducing new models of care entirely within their existing budgets.

The chief registrar programme was another key Commission recommendation. This encapsulates the RCP's aspiration to access the clinical and workforce insights of junior doctors and to provide them with tools to catalyse quality improvement and become future health care leaders. Over 12 months, specialist registrars close to training completion spend two days a week acquiring skills in quality improvement, management and leadership. The programme, still in its first year, has been widely praised and complements initiatives to enhance the careers and working conditions of junior doctors (Royal College of Physicians 2016a, c).

The RCP also seeks to champion innovative care models elsewhere through its publications, the Future Hospital Programme partners network and the 'Tell us your story' initiative. As Future Hospital Programme development site activity winds down in 2017, the challenge is to scale up the adoption of quality improvement as a means of delivering tangible change, from a handful of clinical sites to every acute trust. The RCP is creating a quality improvement hub, supported by a digitally enabled RCP North in Liverpool, with the aim of disseminating learning and support for quality improvement nationally. This in turn will be augmented by the expanding pool of chief registrar alumni, armed with quality improvement skills and experience.

## Measuring to improve

The next decade will see a critical shift towards generating smart data on the performance of multidisciplinary teams, as heralded in *Using data to improve care* (Royal College of Physicians 2015). The result: a scaling down of measurement for assurance (individual clinicians and organisations) and the scaling up of measurement for improvement. Digital technology will blossom (at last), through tracking and monitoring patients and capturing staff interventions.

Trust performance departments will need to be agile in supporting their clinical teams and knowing exactly what support is needed – from replacing faulty hardware to joining up clunky software. The RCP will have a key role in promoting robust measurement of patient care and weaning boards and regulators off performance reporting methodology, which has little or no statistical value.

The final Future Hospital Programme report, due in late 2017, will evaluate the impact of Future Hospital-aligned interventions on patient care and the effectiveness of the 'hub and spoke' programme delivery model. However, insights into what can be achieved through collaborative working with patients and clinicians are already prompting the RCP to explore a consultancy model designed to support clinical staff and acute trusts. The aim would be to bring together best practice in measurement, quality improvement, staff training and support, alongside setting and maintaining the highest standards of medical care.

## An independent foundation's perspective: Jocelyn Cornwell

*Jocelyn Cornwell is chief executive of The Point of Care Foundation. She originally trained as a medical sociologist and ethnographer before joining the NHS as a community manager. Before founding The Point of Care Foundation, Jocelyn worked in management and regulation in the NHS for more than 30 years.*

What is an acute medical ward for? Who defines its purpose and value?

Instead of the prevailing definition of the ward as a medical workplace, it would be better defined as a place for healing, where people are set on the road to recovery from illness and, when recovery is not possible, where pain and distress can be eased by caring professionals. When value is defined from the supply side alone, by clinicians and managers, it tends to ignore relational and non-clinical aspects of care that are critical to patients' mental and emotional wellbeing and to their recovery.

A broader definition of value would recognise how illness affects patients. Illness disturbs our normal ability to cope; it is unsettling, induces anxiety and fear, and makes us vulnerable. Carel (2007), with experience of a life-threatening, chronic condition, observes:

*Illness changes everything. It changes not only my internal organs, but my relationship to my body, my relationship to others, their relation to me and to my body… In short, illness changes how one is in the world.*

Admission to hospital may bring relief, but it increases that vulnerability. As Sweeney *et al* (2009) describe: 'Every patient that comes through a hospital is apprehensive. It's a strange place, you have strange sheets, you have odd tea in a plastic cup. The whole thing is vibrantly different.'

For patients the hospital environment is always unfamiliar: on admission, they lose their autonomy, their right to move, eat and drink at will, to sleep or wake up and to choose their own company.

This is how McCrum (1998) puts it:

*Being a patient is, as the word implies, totally passive. You are dependent upon the nurses; you are always saying thank you and falling in with nurses' jokey routines. If you don't, you become a 'bad' patient to be punished in all kinds of subtle but unmistakable ways. The point is to be passive and appreciative.*

Adults find themselves dependent on others for help with the most basic issues of hygiene and personal care (McCrum 1998): 'There is a curious intimacy in hospital – nobody has anything to hide. Once you are here, you expose every part of your body to the nurses. There's no privacy. As well as this, you are weak and they are strong.'

Feeling dependent and exposed in this way makes patients constantly aware of the power that (all) staff have over them and makes them acutely sensitive to the feeling and tone of all interactions.

*There is nothing funny about clutching a plastic bag with all your clothes in, except your pants, socks, and shoes […] while trying to secure a hospital gown around you, and following, like some faithful gun dog, a radiology attendant who without introduction commands you, with a broad grin to acknowledge his witty lack of grammar, to 'follow I!'*
(Sweeney *et al* 2009)

*A patient was moved opposite my father. He was extremely poorly and it was apparent that he was close to passing away. We were unable to close our curtains to allow him and his family some dignity and privacy, as the nurses needed to see our monitor. We all felt extremely uncomfortable and devastated for the poor family who were all there saying their goodbyes with a whole ward full of people surrounding them with no privacy.*

(Anonymous, daughter, The Point of Care Foundation website)

*A doctor who attended my father [...] was extremely rude. They had been told that my father needed hourly checks but this wasn't happening on the Sunday. When my mum mentioned this to the doctor she snapped, 'There is no way anyone would have approved that'. It was very unsettling.*

(Anonymous, daughter, The Point of Care Foundation website)

Staff do not intend patients to suffer, far from it, but patients are inadvertently exposed to shame and humiliation; to distress, when their requests are ignored or overridden; to anxiety, about being kept in the dark, and about discontinuities and contradictory information; and to fear, when they are unable to trust caregivers.

If wards were defined as places for healing, recovery and care, staff would aim to reduce and eliminate all avoidable suffering (Lee 2015). The quality of relational care would have equal priority to clinical quality and patient safety, and changes in the physical environment, the conduct of staff and the organisation of care would follow.

Staff would be aware of themselves as 'on stage' when in sight or earshot of patients and visitors, and act accordingly. They would always introduce themselves by name and explain their role to new patients (Hello my name is... 2017). They would welcome visitors and involve them where possible. They would sit down to talk, would listen more, would be curious about patients' wants and needs and would strive to have equal discussions about the goals of treatment. They would ask permission before touching the patient's body and share information about the patient as a person with colleagues. They would trust managers to support them when they made changes to benefit patients and to act on their concerns about anything in the physical environment, relationships with colleagues or resources that could be detrimental for patients.

The managers' primary task would be to enable staff to be at their best and to deliver the best care possible. They would know that patients are always at risk because the familiarity staff have with the physical environment and with work routines inevitably blunts their awareness of patients' sensitivities. Managers would be sure to spend time on the wards themselves to observe staff interacting with patients.

They would look for evidence of human touches in patients' care and see their absence as red flags, signals that the team climate might need attention. They would make sure that staff had access to patient feedback and were equipped with the tools and techniques – such as observations of care and patient shadowing – that would refresh their awareness of the patients' experiences and enable them to make improvements (The Point of Care Foundation 2016). They would be aware of how staff use their time, would help them reduce time-wasting activities and insist on them observing breaks and leaving the ward in their rest periods (NHS Improving Quality 2017).

The executive team would not leave the quality of relational care to chance but would see its role as identifying the systemic obstacles to good relational and clinical care, and then dismantle them. They would aim to protect and increase the time that frontline staff spend with patients, by radically reducing the administrative load on the wards and culling top-down demands for information. Accepting that surveys have their limitations, they would equip themselves with multiple sources of intelligence about the quality of care and actively seek out patients and staff to hear their views and opinions (Dixon-Woods *et al* 2014).

They would invest in developing the people skills of frontline managers, and offer all staff opportunities for reflective practice and self-care (The Point of Care Foundation, undated). They would keep staffing levels, staff engagement and staff wellbeing under review, and seek to delegate as much control down the line as possible. Finally, they would invite patients and families to contribute to definitions of value, and ask them to collaborate in service design and improvement and to participate as equals, alongside the professionals, in the workings of the hospital.

# ④ Conclusion

## Bringing it all together: Chris Ham and Don Berwick

The essays in this report offer a range of perspectives on frontline clinical care in acute hospitals. They draw on the experience of staff and patients to shine a light on aspects of NHS care that are often hidden from view. In this conclusion, we summarise the key messages and outline what needs to happen to support staff and improve patient care.

We begin by highlighting the increasing intensity of clinical work. We then proceed into a summary of some of the solutions being developed within the NHS and other health care systems. We conclude by seeking to clarify the role of managers, clinicians, professional societies, regulators, government and patients in bringing about improvements in care.

In writing this conclusion, we wish to emphasise that the challenge of delivering safe and high-quality care at the front line is not new to the NHS. Divisions within medicine and between medicine and other clinical professions have long been recognised as barriers to teamworking. Changes to medical training have added new obstacles. Sustained financial constraints and growth in the demand for care have brought these issues to a head.

Elin Roddy, Michael Wise, Jocelyn Cornwell and other contributors provide eloquent testimony of how these issues are experienced by staff and patients. Their experiences have been underlined by the Care Quality Commission's (CQC) assessment of safety and quality in hospitals across England, just published as we were finishing this report (Care Quality Commission 2017). Our hope is that the voices of staff and patients in this report will enable the longstanding challenges outlined here and by CQC to be addressed with new urgency.

### Pressures at the front line of care

The work that lies behind this report has made us ever more aware of the growing intensity of clinical work as increasing demand for care collides with resource constraints. Clinical teams inside and outside hospitals have acted as 'shock absorbers' in a system that is stretched to and sometimes beyond its limits (Ham 2016b). How long this can continue is unknowable, but the toll is high both on patient care and on staff delivering that care.

Clinical teams in hospitals experience this growing intensity as a demand on them to care for more patients than they feel is possible with the resources at their disposal. We heard accounts of doctors, nurses and other staff not being able to spend sufficient time with each patient and being forced to cut corners. In some areas of care, workload pressures are compounded by requirements to meet externally imposed targets that may distort clinical priorities.

Although there are no agreed standards for the number of acutely ill medical patients who can safely be seen by a consultant physician and his or her team, we perceive a consensus that the current volume is at the outer limit of feasibility. This is particularly the case when patients have complex needs that require time and expertise of different kinds to resolve and when the quality of decision-making may be affected by the amount of work to be done. The patient stories in this report confirm that safety is sometimes put at risk in these circumstances.

Increasing reliance on agency staff and gaps in staff rotas accentuate the difficulties in providing the effective continuity and teamwork on which good care in today's NHS depends. Michael Wise cites an example from his experience of agency staff who were not aware of the requirements of a transplant patient. Multidisciplinary ward rounds do not always include the full range of staff involved in patient care and this adds to the pressures on doctors. Junior doctors find themselves under strain when they are required to cover gaps in staffing and may not have timely access to senior advice and support (Royal College of Physicians 2016a).

Workload pressures are a source of stress for staff as well as compromising the quality of patient care. The demands placed on clinical teams are leading to higher levels of sickness absence, compounding staffing gaps. Work stress may also cause some staff to leave the NHS for less pressurised environments in health care or other sectors. Staff shortages across the NHS suggest this is already causing problems.

Difficulties in recruiting doctors to acute medicine – with 44 per cent of advertised consultant posts unfilled in 2016 – mean that there are insufficient numbers of specialists to meet growing demand for care. Recruitment is especially challenging in acute internal medicine and geriatric medicine. These are two of the specialties most involved in the care of the acutely ill medical patients who are the focus of this report (Royal College of Physicians 2016b).

Seven years of historically low levels of growth in NHS funding coupled with workforce shortages are making it difficult to maintain current standards of care – let alone assure continual improvement. Their effects have been amplified by fast-rising demand for care (Maguire *et al* 2016). Cuts in publicly funded social care have added to the pressures on the NHS as seen in increasing numbers of hospital patients waiting to be discharged.

We fully recognise that the NHS budget has received greater protection than other public services in recent years at a time when public finances have been constrained, and this is to be welcomed. Yet despite the commitment of additional resources, NHS spending as a share of national income is now on a downward trend and per capita spending on health care is also falling (Emmerson *et al* 2017). Unless the government is willing to increase planned spending on the NHS and social care and to address workforce shortages, pressures on patients and staff will become even greater, and perhaps unsustainable.

## Solutions being developed within the NHS

Under these circumstances, it is heartening that many clinical teams, with support from trust leaders, are finding solutions to some of the challenges we have described. These solutions include Northumbria's joining up information systems to give clinical teams access to patients' records in different settings; the use of board rounds alongside ward rounds in Sandwell and West Birmingham and other hospitals; and improvements in handover arrangements between shifts at the Royal Free to strengthen communication between staff and improve continuity of care for patients.

An increasing number of trusts are investing in quality improvement programmes in their own organisations. In the essays in this report, Imperial College, Sheffield and Western Sussex are good examples. Each has made a commitment to training and supporting staff to use scientifically grounded quality improvement methods to identify problems and then test and implement solutions. They do so by 'going to the gemba' and by exploiting the cumulative impact of many small changes over time. Patient-flow projects in Sheffield and other hospitals and the redesigned emergency floor in Western Sussex illustrate what this means.

Other solutions are being tested through the Future Hospital Programme run by the Royal College of Physicians (RCP) and the new care models programme. One of the insights from the RCP's work is the value of focusing on early assessment and early discharge of medical patients admitted as emergencies to avoid problems further down the track. These problems often arise when patients are moved between wards instead of having their conditions diagnosed and dealt with promptly. Promising early reports from the hospitals participating in this programme illustrate the potential benefits of such an approach.

The new care models programme set up to implement the NHS five year forward view is supporting hospitals to work more closely with general practices, community services and social care (NHS England 2016). Effective co-operative processes can help prevent patients being admitted to acute hospitals or remaining in hospitals longer than necessary by providing alternative services in the community, including intermediate care. Whole-system redesign of this kind holds out the promise of reducing demands on hospitals and specialists through more fundamental improvements than are feasible within hospitals alone.

New partnerships between GPs and specialists are developing in some of the new care model sites. These partnerships have the potential to bridge the gap described by Rammya Mathew and John Launer in their contribution to this report – for example, by making it easier for GPs to seek the advice of specialists through secure email links. James O'Brien's essay shows how a telephone hotline and a 'hot clinic' for children has improved communication between GPs and specialists in one trust.

## Junior doctors as agents of improvement

Frontline staff almost invariably seek to meet rising patient demands and when they fall short, it is usually because of defects in the systems in which they operate and lack of staff and resources. As Bob Klaber emphasises in his essay, critically important to successful redesign and improvement is adopting the right tone –

one in which clinical staff feel valued and respected. This includes listening to staff and acting on their insights, which often hold the key to unlocking improvements in care.

It also means avoiding the stereotyping and professional insularity observed by Harrison Carter in his essay by moving beyond the hierarchies and tribal divisions that are longstanding barriers to teamworking. Effective medical and surgical care requires high-functioning teams, and all members have a part to play in both delivering and improving care. Junior doctors are particularly valuable because of their ability to compare and contrast practices in different hospitals through the rotations they undertake during training.

The challenge, described well in several essays in this report, is that too few organisations appear to seek and value junior doctors' insights, a view confirmed in other reports (Goddard 2017). The knowledge of medical students and junior doctors is 'gold dust', and should be mined relentlessly. This is best done hospital by hospital but needs to be supported by national leaders showing respect for and valuing the critical contribution of the workforce of the future and by demonstrating that they understand the realities of care at the front line.

We heard how changes in the training of junior doctors within the NHS are having undesired side effects. The move away from the 'firm' model, in which junior doctors were attached to a medical team during training, has resulted in a more fragmented experience for these doctors. Reductions in the working hours of junior doctors and the move to four-month rotations, rather than six months, add to the sense of fragmentation. Building and maintaining relationships with senior medical colleagues and other clinicians appears to be more difficult than ever.

One of the consequences of changes in training is that senior medical students have fewer opportunities than previously to develop skills in clinical procedures and to gain experience of clinical decision-making. This is compounded by hospital consultants taking on greater responsibility as 'senior review' of patients becomes more frequent to deal with growing pressures on beds and increasing patient complexity. These changes contribute to the dissatisfaction expressed by junior doctors who may have less opportunity to practise autonomously (Oliver 2017).

Changes in medical training contribute to high rates of stress among doctors in training and to increased sickness rates (Campbell 2017; Royal College of Physicians 2016a). These issues have been simmering for some time and were brought to the boil by the dispute over the new contract for junior doctors. Goddard has argued that declining morale among these doctors results from a combination of substantial workloads, loss of team structure, poor quality training, and lack of flexibility in working arrangements (Goddard 2016).

Surveys of junior doctors underline the importance of creating working environments that enable all staff, including trainees, to practise to the best of their abilities, and to experience joy and pride in their work. The chief executive of NHS England, Simon Stevens, has acknowledged that this issue needs to be addressed. Some NHS trusts, such as Birmingham Women's and Children's Hospitals, have listened to the concerns of junior doctors and have changed ways of working to create a more supportive and stimulating environment in which to provide care (West *et al* 2017).

## Collaboration and co-ordination

Collaboration and co-ordination are essential if patients are to receive the best possible care. Staff need to have sufficient time to care and to co-ordinate the treatment of patients who often have complex medical conditions that can be difficult to diagnose and treat. Press (2014) has written about these issues in the US context, arguing that the physician has a key role in co-ordinating the contribution of the increasing number of clinicians involved in treating patients with complex needs.

Care co-ordination is a patient safety issue because 'patients can be harmed when the many moving parts of their care are out of sync' (Press 2014, p 489). Press argues that teamwork 'must encompass multiple clinical settings, where team members might not see or know each other' (p 490). This requires systems designed to facilitate collaboration, for example through sharing information about patients and allowing time for communication among clinicians. In the absence of these possibilities, there is a risk of the 'bystander effect' (Stavert and Lott 2013), which occurs when clinicians involved in a patient's care may not intervene because responsibility is shared with others and it is unclear who is in charge.

Collaboration and co-ordination are dependent on clinicians having well-developed relationships with each other and opportunities to build these relationships. This is often challenging in the NHS both within acute hospitals and among hospitals, GPs and others involved in providing care, such as transferring hospitals. Solutions centre on finding ways for clinicians to meet and talk to each other to build the connections and understandings on which good care depends.

Collaboration and co-ordination are critically dependent on doctors and other clinicians having time to communicate with colleagues about patients. The growing intensity of clinical work in acute hospitals makes it difficult to do this when the immediate pressures of diagnosing, treating and discharging patients take precedence. The job plans of hospital doctors caring for acutely ill medical patients must build in time for communicating with hospital colleagues, GPs and others to avoid safety being compromised. Staffing shortages are a barrier to this happening and cultures of care are also important (*see* below).

Steve Swensen of Mayo Clinic emphasises the importance of 'commensality' – time to eat and talk together – in relationship building (Ham 2016a). Surveys of doctors in training show how these human issues are often neglected with lack of access to food and water and breaks being common concerns (Royal College of Physicians 2016a). Paying attention to these issues is essential to address rising discontent among junior doctors and to establish the relationships on which collaboration and co-ordination depend.

## Standardisation of care and systems

The revolution needed in health care delivery requires clinicians to move from being skilled, individual craftsmen and craftswomen to becoming enthusiastic members of teams that deliver care consistently in line with evidence-based guidelines and, when appropriate, standardised processes (Swensen *et al* 2010). This entails planning and specifying how clinical work is done at a level of detail that hitherto has been confined to only a few areas of medical practice and a small number of health care systems such as Intermountain Healthcare in the United States (Bohmer 2009). In many health care systems, clinical autonomy remains a barrier to the adoption of standardised processes even when there is evidence that such processes improve safety and the quality of care.

Gawande has drawn an unlikely parallel between hospitals and the Cheesecake Factory restaurant chain to make this point. He describes how the restaurant business plans and specifies the introduction of new menus through training staff in kitchens and front-of-house in a way that leaves little to chance. By extension he argues that in health care, 'we're moving from a Jeffersonian ideal of small guilds and independent craftsmen to a Hamiltonian recognition of the advantages that size and centralised control can bring' (Gawande 2012). In his view, this requires recognition that good medical care results from the system in which clinical teams deliver this care.

The system to which Gawande is referring encompasses both the environment in which care is delivered (such as buildings and IT) and processes that clinical teams use to care for patients. These processes include the conduct of ward rounds, the allocation of responsibilities among different team members, availability of information to support decision-making, and relationships with clinicians in other parts of the hospital, other hospitals, GPs, and community resources including social care. The design of these processes – and indeed whether they are designed or have evolved through custom and practice – shape how the components of care work together to deliver the best possible outcomes.

Sam Pannick is another author who argues for greater standardisation to counter what he describes as the 'arbitrary' way in which ward rounds, board rounds and multidisciplinary meetings are organised in the NHS. In his view, the five elements of care that matter most on wards are team composition, interdisciplinary collaboration, care standardisation, early treatment of the deteriorating patient, and local safety climate. Sam contends that a continuous focus on the operational aspects of care delivery and how they can be standardised is the route to improvement. He argues that ward care should be prioritised as an organisational objective and concludes by stating: 'We need to be much harder on our systems: this will help us to be far, far kinder to our people.'

Sam is here echoing Bohmer's work that makes the case for the 'operating systems' of clinical care to be given much more attention (Bohmer 2016, 2010). Although the design of these operating systems has received insufficient attention in the NHS, there are examples of work that can be used to support progress. In the case of the acutely ill medical patients who are the focus of this report, the Emergency Care Intensive Support Team has produced advice and guidance based on experience in

4

different parts of the NHS. This includes ensuring early senior review of patients, putting patients on the right pathways and improving discharge planning (NHS Improvement 2017).

The challenge is to act systematically on these and similar examples across the NHS. If this does not happen, there is a risk that unco-ordinated local quality improvement projects will make it more difficult to standardise care across the NHS (Dixon-Woods and Pronovost 2016).

## Cultures of care

While standardisation is undoubtedly important, no amount of planning and specification of how clinical work should be done can substitute for organisational cultures in which 'the needs of the patient come first' (to borrow from Mayo Clinic). Among other things, this means avoiding the desensitisation of staff that can harm patients, however inadvertently, as noted by Michael Wise in his contribution to this report. If culture, at its simplest, is 'the way things are done round here', then this has to be worked on continuously to ensure that it really does focus on patients (Awdish 2017).

Jocelyn Cornwell reminds us in her contribution that the hospital ward is not only a place of work but also, and above all, 'a place for healing, where people incapacitated by illness are set on the road to recovery, and if recovery is not possible, where pain and distress are eased by caring professionals'. As Clare Carter-Jones observes, this requires open-mindedness and insight to understand that what may appear good care to those providing it may be experienced quite differently by those receiving the care and by their families. Whatever the pressures faced by staff as workloads increase, professionalism demands that patients should always be the focus of care.

Developing and nurturing caring cultures must start at the top with senior hospital leaders centring their own decisions and actions on the needs of the patient. Survey data and active solicitation of the voices of patients, carers and staff can help leaders to understand the extent to which the focus on needs is succeeding. Observations of care and patient shadowing, as used in the patient and family-centred care programme (The King's Fund 2014), have a part to play in this process. Mike Richards notes in his contribution that a passion for high-quality patient-centred care is one of the characteristics of outstanding NHS trusts.

The tragic events at Mid Staffordshire NHS Foundation Trust illustrate what happens when cultures of this kind are not in place. They are a reminder, if one were needed, of why attending to the experience of patients as well as frontline clinical staff is so important. The recommendations of the Berwick report, set up in response to the inquiry into Mid Staffordshire, provide a framework on what the NHS should do to become a learning organisation committed to improving the safety of patients (National Advisory Group on the Safety of Patients in England 2013).

## Managers and clinicians

The leaders of NHS trusts, with some exceptions, have not been able to find the time to focus systematically on improving the operating systems through which care is organised at the front line. This is partly because they have been preoccupied with responding to the demands of the regulators but it also reflects the clinical autonomy of hospital specialists dating back to the origins of the NHS (Klein 2010). Many trust leaders also lack training and skills in quality improvement and may not have access to the resources to acquire such skills.

Variations in clinical care are a predictable consequence of a system that emphasises clinical autonomy at the expense of reliability (Briggs 2015). Tackling these variations requires systematic measurement of how care is delivered, as Mike Durkin argues in his essay, and leaders who are confident in using data to challenge clinicians to make improvements. It also requires clinical leaders who are able to work with trust leaders and clinicians in reducing unwarranted variations in care.

Leaders in high-performing organisations such as the Virginia Mason Medical Center (VMMC) stand out because they make a deep and continuing personal commitment to quality improvement. Marianne Griffiths, chief executive of Western Sussex Hospitals NHS Foundation Trust, has described to us her epiphany in learning about the work of the VMMC, and the impact on her leadership style. This included learning to trust and support staff to make improvements in care and resisting the temptation to intervene when problems emerge.

Marianne is clear that a commitment to quality improvement is quite different from the 'turnaround' programmes typically used to support NHS trusts that get into difficulty. She goes further to argue that being in turnaround makes it all nigh impossible to make the changes on which sustained improvement rests because leaders are distracted by the demands of the regulators. Because Western Sussex was not preoccupied with dealing with requests from the regulators, it therefore had the time and opportunity to commit to the Patients First programme (*see* Introduction).

The development of clinical leadership from the Griffiths Report (1983) onwards has been important in bringing clinical expertise into leadership teams, both at the trust level and in the divisions and directorates through which services are organised. Medical and nursing directors and their clinical colleagues in other leadership roles now play a key part in managing hospitals and in working with frontline teams to improve how their work is done. These teams are able to draw on national improvement programmes like the productive ward initiative as well as trust-based improvement programmes such as those described in this report.

Clinical leaders at trust level and in other roles have a particular responsibility to lead quality improvement work, as several of the essays in this report illustrate. The role of these leaders is to signal their commitment to improvements in care through their actions, words, investments and behaviours, and through what they attend to. George Findlay, medical director at Western Sussex, explained to us how he spends time 'in the gemba', coaching the members of clinical teams in their efforts to improve care. Salford Royal NHS Foundation Trust is another organisation in which the executive team works in this way (Ham 2014).

An example from Western Sussex on how this is done is a standing-up meeting in a clinical area, open to the public, with staff in the intensive therapy unit (ITU). The meeting uses improvement methodology and visual displays to support problem solving in which all relevant staff are involved. The focus is delayed discharge from ITU, which is a poor use of expensive critical care facilities and not usually a way of delivering optimal patient care. George and his colleagues in the trust's executive team are able to work in this way because they make themselves available to staff who are delivering care.

At Western Sussex, the trust's leaders are visible to staff and demonstrate what matters by how they spend their time and where they work. Both George Findlay and Marianne Griffiths emphasise that they are more effective when they avoid, in their words, 'putting the cape on' in the style of superman or superwoman to intervene directly, and instead stand back to allow clinical staff to find solutions. Divisional and clinical directors in the trust are encouraged to work in a similar way. Being visible at the front line and supporting staff to improve care is part of the commitment to good clinical governance in the trust.

Yet even in NHS trusts that have embraced quality improvement, middle managers in hospitals are preoccupied with maintaining existing services and supporting teams to deal with intense operational pressures, as illustrated in the contributions by Juliet Shavin and James O'Brien. Writing from a GP perspective Rammya Mathew and John Launer describe the sense of firefighting that occurs in crowded hospital environments. Firefighting is also how many clinicians encounter care, as illustrated by the experience reported by Elin Roddy.

Gordon Caldwell describes clinicians as 'hunter gatherers' who are constantly chasing information about patients rather than having it readily available. Jennifer Isherwood recounts the time spent in finding patients who may have moved wards, an experience all too common in the NHS and one that David Oliver has likened to going on safari (Oliver 2016). The dilemma for clinicians and managers, as Elin Roddy notes, is that finding the time to tackle the causes of these frustrations would mean using time that would otherwise be spent caring for patients.

Middle managers could play an important part in improving how care is organised to address these and other challenges if they had the time and resources to do so. One of the reasons they often do not do so is that the health care sector in England has been slow to take up quality improvement methods that have contributed to process improvements and standardisation in other industries (Ham *et al* 2016). The NHS needs to embrace quality improvement across the entire sector, focusing on organisational strengthening, and building capacity for improvement, and not take a piecemeal, project-based approach (Dixon-Woods and Martin 2016). This should build on the contribution of organisations like the Health Foundation and others with expertise to offer.

The NHS also needs to recognise the joint responsibility of clinicians and managers to join up their efforts to improve care, supported by professional societies and organisations with quality improvement expertise (Ham and Alberti 2002). Clinicians have a responsibility to advise managers of the support they need and should be willing to recognise that established habits and processes may not be delivering care safely and efficiently. Hospital leaders and those in middle management roles should visibly support clinicians to improve care in organisationally led improvement efforts of the kind found in Western Sussex and Salford Royal. Working relentlessly to bridge the gap between executive teams and those delivering and organising care at the front line must be the priority in every NHS trust.

## We're all in this together

We began this report by asking where responsiblity for improving clinical care at the front line should rest. Our answer is that it should be everybody's responsibility, from the clinical teams delivering care through leaders of NHS trusts and onwards to professional societies, national regulators, government and patients. Leaders of local systems of care, such as those being developed in Sustainability and Transformation Plans, can help by redesigning care through new care models that support patients to flow into and out of hospitals more effectively, and to avoid hospital admission where appropriate. No stakeholder ought to be a bystander.

National regulators including CQC, Health Education England, NHS England and NHS Improvement have a part to play in providing oversight of how clinical care is organised and the resources to support good care. This includes resources to modernise physical space, equipment and information technology, as well as to train and develop the workforce of the future. The latter includes the use of new roles such as physician associates where appropriate. Government has a responsibility to provide sufficient and sustainable funding to enable staff to meet rising patient demands safely and effectively.

National regulators should change fundamentally their approach to supporting trusts that have performance challenges. External support of the kind provided by management consultants should be replaced with a commitment to quality improvement led by NHS leaders with a track record of delivering change. This means valuing and trusting staff, listening to their concerns, and creating the headroom for frontline clinical teams to improve the care for which they are responsible.

The experience of organisations where this has happened provides compelling evidence of the benefits of this way of working. This evidence shows what can happen when the NHS reforms itself 'from within' by joining expertise at the front line with the commitment of NHS trust leaders (Ham 2014). It is a reminder that the primary responsibility for the provision of safe and high-quality care rests with the teams providing this care, while trust leaders and national regulators provide the second and third lines of defence (Dixon *et al* 2012). This is the essence of the modern definition of professionalism described in our introduction.

Our hope is that this report, as the first product of an appreciative inquiry into frontline clinical care, will draw attention to the experience of staff and patients in an NHS that is facing unprecedented pressures. We urge managers and clinicians to pay more attention to the organisation of care at the front line and work together to remove the barriers that get in the way of care being provided safely every time. We call on the government to be honest about the impact of financial pressures on staff and patients and on national regulators to change their approach to performance management and improvement. Everyone involved in the NHS should commit to putting the needs of the patient first.

We invite readers to get involved by contributing their experiences and ideas on the solutions that are needed.

# References

Awdish RLA (2017). 'A view from the edge – creating a culture of caring'. *New England Journal of Medicine*, vol 376, pp 7–9.

Bohmer RM (2016). 'The hard work of health care transformation'. *New England Journal of Medicine*, vol 375, pp 709–11.

Bohmer R (2010). 'Fixing health care on the front lines'. *Harvard Business Review*. Available at: https://hbr.org/2010/04/fixing-health-care-on-the-front-lines (accessed on 9 March 2017).

Bohmer R (2009). *Designing care: aligning the nature and management of health care*. Boston: Harvard Business Press.

Briggs T (2015). *A national review of adult elective orthopaedic services in England: getting it right first time*. British Orthopaedic Association. Available at: www.boa.ac.uk/wp-content/uploads/2015/03/GIRFT-National-Report-MarN.pdf (accessed on 9 March 2017).

Burnett S, Franklin BD, Moorthy K, Cooke MW, Vincent C (2012). 'How reliable are clinical systems in the UK NHS? A study of seven NHS organisations'. *British Medical Journal Quality and Safety*, vol 21, pp 466–72.

Campbell D (2017). 'Most young doctors "suffering burnout"'. *The Observer*, 12 Feb.

Carel H (2007). 'My 10-year death sentence'. *Independent* website. Available at: www.independent.co.uk/news/people/profiles/havi-carel-my-10-year-death-sentence-5332425.html (accessed on 24 February 2017).

Care Quality Commission (2017). *The state of care in NHS acute hospitals: 2014 to 2016*. Findings from the end of CQC's programme of NHS acute comprehensive inspections. Available at: www.cqc.org.uk/content/state-care-nhs-acute-hospitals (accessed on 9 March 2017).

Care Quality Commission (2016). 'Provider handbooks'. CQC website. Available at: www.cqc.org.uk/content/provider-handbooks (accessed on 20 March 2017).

Department of Health (2008). *High quality care for all: NHS Next Stage final report*. Cm: 7432. London: The Stationery Office. Available at: www.gov.uk/government/publications/high-quality-care-for-all-nhs-next-stage-review-final-report (accessed on 14 March 2017).

Department of Health Expert Group (2000). *An organisation with a memory: report of an expert group on learning from adverse events in the NHS*. Chair: Sir Liam Donaldson. London: The

Stationery Office. Available at: http://webarchive.nationalarchives.gov.uk/20130107105354/http://www.dh.gov.uk/en/Publicationsandstatistics/Publications/PublicationsPolicyAndGuidance/DH_4065083 (accessed on 14 March 2017).

Dixon A, Foot C, Harrison T (2012). *Preparing for the Francis Report: how to assure quality in the NHS*. London: The King's Fund. Available at: www.kingsfund.org.uk/publications/articles/preparing-francis-report-how-assure-quality-nhs (accessed on 15 March 2017).

Dixon-Woods M, Martin GP (2016). 'Does quality improvement improve quality?'. *Future Hospital Journal*, vol 3, no 3, pp 191–4.

Dixon-Woods M, Provonost P (2016). 'Patient safety and the problem of many hands.' *BMJ Quality and Safety*, vol 25, pp 485–8. Available at: http://qualitysafety.bmj.com/content/25/7/485 (Accessed on 10 April 2017).

Dixon-Woods M, Baker R, Charles K, Dawson J, Jerzembek G, Martin G, McCarthy I, McKee L, Minion J, Ozieranski P, Willars J, Wilkie P, West M (2014). 'Culture and behaviour in the English National Health Service: overview of lessons from a large multimethod study'. *BMJ Quality and Safety*, vol 23, pp 106–15. Available at: http://qualitysafety.bmj.com/content/23/2/106 (accessed on 14 March 2017).

Emmerson C, Johnson P, Joyce R (2017). 'IFS green budget 2017'. Institute for Fiscal Studies website. Available at: www.ifs.org.uk/publications/8825 (accessed on 9 March 2017).

Future Hospital Commission (2013). *Future hospital: caring for medical patients* [online]. Royal College of Physicians website. Available at: www.rcplondon.ac.uk/projects/outputs/future-hospital-commission (accessed on 24 February 2017).

Gawande A (2012). 'Big med: restaurant chains have managed to combine quality control, cost control and innovation. Can health care?'. *The New Yorker*. Available at: www.newyorker.com/magazine/2012/08/13/big-med (accessed on 9 March 2017).

Goddard A (2017). 'Whither or wither the medical registrar?'. *Future Hospital Journal*, vol 4, no 1, pp 39–43.

Goddard A (2016). 'Lessons to be learned from the UK junior doctors' strike'. *Journal of the American Medical Association*, vol 316, no 14, pp 1445–6.

Griffiths R (1983). 'NHS management inquiry'. Letter to Rt Hon Norman Fowler, Secretary of State for Social Services. Available at: www.nhshistory.net/griffiths.html (accessed on 15 March 2017).

Ham C (2016a). 'Commensality – or bring back the lunch break'. Blog. The King's Fund website. Available at: www.kingsfund.org.uk/blog/2016/11/commensality-bring-back-lunch-break (accessed on 9 March 2017).

Ham C (2016b). 'UK government's autumn statement: no relief for NHS and social care in England'. *British Medical Journal,* vol 355: i6382.

Ham C (2014). *Reforming the NHS from within: beyond hierarchy, inspection and markets.* London: The King's Fund. Available at: www.kingsfund.org.uk/time-to-think-differently/publications/reforming-nhs-within (accessed on 17 March 2017).

Ham C, Alberti K (2002). 'The medical profession, the public, and the government'. *British Medical Journal,* vol 324, p 838.

Ham C, Berwick D, Dixon J (2016). *Improving quality in the English NHS: a strategy for action.* London: The King's Fund. Available at: www.kingsfund.org.uk/publications/quality-improvement (accessed on 9 March 2017).

Hellier C, Tully V, Forrest S, Jaggard P, MacRae M, Habicht D, Greene A, Collins K (2015). 'Improving multidisciplinary communication at ward board rounds using video enhanced reflective practice'. *British Medical Journal Quality Improvement Reports,* vol 4, no 1.

Hello my name is… (2017). Hello my name is… website. Available at: http://hellomynameis.org.uk/ (accessed on 24 February 2017).

Institute of Medicine (2000). *Crossing the quality chasm: a new health system for the 21st century.* Washington: National Academy Press.

Klein R (2010). *The new politics of the NHS: from creation to reinvention,* 2nd ed. Oxford: Radcliffe.

Kohn LT, Corrigan JM, Donaldson MS (eds) (2000). *To err is human: building a safer health system.* Washington: National Academy Press.

Lee TH (2015). *An epidemic of empathy in healthcare: how to deliver compassionate, connected patient care that creates a competitive advantage.* Boston: McGraw-Hill Education.

Maguire D, Dunn P, McKenna H (2016). 'How hospital activity in the NHS in England has changed over time'. London: The King's Fund. Available at: www.kingsfund.org.uk/publications/hospital-activity-funding-changes (accessed on 9 March 2017).

McCrum R (1998). *My year off: rediscovering life after a stroke.* London: Picador.

Mullan F (2001). 'A founder of quality assessment encounters a troubled system firsthand.' *Health Affairs*, vol 20, no 1, pp 137–41. Available at: http://content.healthaffairs.org/content/20/1.toc (accessed on 14 March 2017).

National Advisory Group on the Safety of Patients in England (2013). *A promise to learn – a commitment to act: improving the safety of patients in England.* London: Department of Health. Available at: www.gov.uk/government/publications/berwick-review-into-patient-safety (accessed on 9 March 2017).

NHS England (2016). 'New care models: vanguards – developing a blueprint for the future of NHS and care services'. Available at: www.england.nhs.uk/wp-content/uploads/2015/11/new_care_models.pdf (accessed on 9 March 2017).

NHS Improvement (2017). 'Emergency Care Improvement Programme (ECIP). NHS Improvement website. Available at: https://improvement.nhs.uk/improvement-offers/ecip/ (accessed on 20 March 2017).

NHS Improving Quality (2017). 'The productive series. Releasing time to care'. The Productive Series website. Available at: www.theproductives.com/ (accessed on 14 March 2017).

NHS Improving Quality (2016). 'Seven day services clinical standards: revisions to supporting information for seven day services clinical standards 2, 5, and 8'. Slide set. Available at: http://webarchive.nationalarchives.gov.uk/20160506181809/http://www.nhsiq.nhs.uk/media/2638611/clinical_standards.pdf (accessed on 24 February 2017).

Oliver D (2017). 'Is the ward round dead?'. *BMJ*, 2017, 356: j635. Available at: www.bmj.com/content/356/bmj.j635 (accessed on 20 March 2017).

Oliver D (2016). 'Reducing delays in hospital'. *BMJ*, 2016, 354: i5125. Available at: www.bmj.com/content/354/bmj.i5125 (accessed on 20 March 2017).

Pannick S, Sevdalis N, Athanasiou T (2016a). 'Beyond clinical engagement: a pragmatic model for quality improvement interventions, aligning clinical and managerial priorities'. *British Medical Journal Quality and Safety*, vol 25, pp 716–25.

Pannick S, Wachter RM, Vincent C, Sevdalis N (2016b). 'Rethinking medical ward quality.' *BMJ*, vol 55. Available at: www.bmj.com/content/355/bmj.i5417 (accessed on 25 April 2017).

Pannick S, Davis R, Ashrafian H, Byrne BE, Beveridge I, Athanasiou T, Wachter RM, Sevdalis N (2015). 'Effects of interdisciplinary team care interventions on general medical wards: a systematic review'. *JAMA Internal Medicine*, vol 175, pp 1288–98.

Pannick S, Beveridge I, Wachter RM, Sevdalis N (2014). 'Improving the quality and safety of care on the medical ward: a review and synthesis of the evidence base'. *European Journal of Internal Medicine*, vol 25, pp 874–87.

Press J (2014). 'Instant replay – a quarterback's view of care coordination'. *New England Journal of Medicine,* vol 371, pp 489–91.

Royal College of Physicians (2016a). *Being a junior doctor* [online]. Royal College of Physicians website. Available at: www.rcplondon.ac.uk/guidelines-policy/being-junior-doctor (accessed on 24 February 2017).

Royal College of Physicians (2016b). *Focus on physicians: census of consultant physicians and higher specialty trainees 2015–16.* Available at: www.rcplondon.ac.uk/projects/outputs/2015-16-census-uk-consultants-and-higher-specialty-trainees (accessed on 9 March 2017).

Royal College of Physicians (2016c). *Keeping medicine brilliant: improving working conditions in acute settings* [online]. Royal College of Physicians website. Available at: www.rcplondon.ac.uk/guidelines-policy/keeping-medicine-brilliant (accessed on 24 February 2017).

Royal College of Physicians (2016d). *Underfunded, underdoctored, overstretched: the NHS in 2016* [online]. Royal College of Physicians website. Available at: www.rcplondon.ac.uk/guidelines-policy/underfunded-underdoctored-overstretched-nhs-2016 (accessed on 24 February 2017).

Royal College of Physicians (2015). *Acute care toolkit no 11: using data to improve care* [online]. Royal College of Physicians website. Available at: www.rcplondon.ac.uk/guidelines-policy/acute-care-toolkit-11-using-data-improve-care (accessed on 24 February 2017).

Royal College of Physicians (2012). *Hospitals on the edge? The time for action* [online]. Royal College of Physicians website. Available at: www.rcplondon.ac.uk/guidelines-policy/hospitals-edge-time-action (accessed on 24 February 2017).

Royal College of Physicians, Royal College of Nursing (2012). *Ward rounds in medicine: principles for best practice* [online]. Royal College of Physicians website. Available at: www.rcplondon.ac.uk/projects/outputs/ward-rounds-medicine-principles-best-practice (accessed on 24 February 2017).

Spear S (2017). *Fast discovery: the imperative for high-velocity learning by everyone, about everything, all of the time.* London: The Health Foundation. Available at: www.health.org.uk/publication/fast-discovery (accessed on 24 February 2017).

Stavert R, Lott J (2013). 'The bystander effect in medical care'. *New England Journal of Medicine,* vol 368, pp 8–9.

Sweeney K, Toy E, Cornwell J (2009). 'A patient's journey. Mesothelioma'. *British Medical Journal,* 2009, 339: b2862 doi: 10.1136/BMJ.b2862

Swensen S, Meyer G, Nelson E, Hunt Jr GC, Pryor DB, Weissberg JI, Kaplan GS, Daley J, Yates GR, Chassin MR, James BC, Berwick DM (2010). 'Cottage industry to postindustrial care – the revolution in health care delivery'. *New England Journal of Medicine,* vol 362, e12.

The King's Fund (2014). 'What is PFCC and why is it needed?.' The King's Fund website. Available at: www.kingsfund.org.uk/projects/pfcc/what-pfcc-and-why-it-needed (accessed on 10 April 2017).

The Point of Care Foundation (2016). *Patient and family-centred care (PFCC) toolkit.* Point of Care Foundation website. Available at: www.pointofcarefoundation.org.uk/resource/patient-family-centred-care-toolkit/ (accessed on 6 March 2017)

The Point of Care Foundation (undated). 'Schwartz Rounds'. The Point of Care Foundation website. Available at www.pointofcarefoundation.org.uk/our-work/schwartz-rounds/ (accessed on 6 March 2017).

Tucker AL (2004). 'The impact of operational failures on hospital nurses and their patients'. *Journal of Operations Management*, vol 22, pp 151–69.

Weick K, Sutcliffe K (2001). *Managing the unexpected: assuring high performance in an sage of complexity.* New Jersey: Wiley, Jossey Bass.

West M, Eckert R, Collins B, Chowla R (2017). *Caring to change: how compassionate leadership can stimulate innovation in health care.* London The King's Fund.

Wise M (2017). *On the toss of a coin.* Leicester: Troubadour.

# About the editors

**Chris Ham** leads the work of The King's Fund. He rejoined the Fund in 2010, having previously worked here between 1986 and 1992. He has held posts at the universities of Birmingham, Bristol and Leeds and is currently emeritus professor at the University of Birmingham. He is an honorary fellow of the Royal College of Physicians of London and the Royal College of General Practitioners.

Chris was director of the strategy unit in the Department of Health between 2000 and 2004, has advised the WHO and the World Bank, and has acted as a consultant to a number of governments. He has been a non-executive director of the Heart of England NHS Foundation Trust, and a governor of the Health Foundation and the Canadian Health Services Research Foundation.

Chris researches and writes on all aspects of health reform and is a sought-after speaker. He was awarded a CBE in 2004 for his services to the NHS and an honorary doctorate by the University of Kent in 2012.

**Don Berwick** became an international visiting fellow at The King's Fund in 2015 and contributes to the Fund's broader work to improve health and care in the NHS.

Don works widely with governmental and non-governmental organisations throughout England as part of his efforts in support of improvement of care, outcomes and costs within the NHS in England.

A paediatrician by background, Don was the founding chief executive of the Institute for Healthcare Improvement for 19 years. In 2010, he was appointed Administrator of the Centers for Medicare and Medicaid Services (the federal agency overseeing Medicare and Medicaid), a position that he held until December 2011. He has served on the faculties of the Harvard Medical School and Harvard School of Public Health.

In 2013 he carried out a review of patient safety in the NHS on behalf of Prime Minister David Cameron. Recognised as a leading authority on health care quality and improvement, Don has authored or co-authored more than 160 scientific articles and six books.

# Acknowledgements

We are indebted to many people who contributed their ideas and insights to the work that lies behind this report. Special thanks are due to Marianne Griffiths and her colleagues at Western Sussex Hospitals NHS Foundation Trust for inviting us to visit and learn from their experience and being generous with their time. Gordon Caldwell allowed us privileged access to his ward round and opened our eyes to the challenges he and colleagues face in providing clinical care in today's NHS. Our fellow authors were enthusiastic in taking up our invitation to contribute their perspectives on the puzzle we encountered at Worthing Hospital and gracious in responding to our requests and suggestions during the editing process. Many others helped guide and educate us in our inquiry. We are particularly grateful to David Oliver who kindly commented on earlier drafts and forced us to clarify our thinking on several points. Participants at the two roundtables we organised offered invaluable confirmation and challenge as the work progressed. Within The King's Fund, we received great support from Laura Carter, Katie Mantell and Lisa Oxlade. Colleagues at NHS England and NHS Improvement worked with us to enable Don to spend time with leaders in the new care models programme which indirectly led to our interest in the issues discussed in this report. We are responsible for any errors or omissions.

**Published by**
The King's Fund
11-13 Cavendish Square
London W1G 0AN
Tel: 020 7307 2568
Fax: 020 7307 2801

Email:
publications@kingsfund.org.uk

www.kingsfund.org.uk

© The King's Fund 2017

First published 2017 by
The King's Fund

Charity registration number:
1126980

All rights reserved, including
the right of reproduction in
whole or in part in any form

ISBN: 978 1 909029 72 9

A catalogue record for this
publication is available from
the British Library

Edited by Anna Brown

Typeset by Peter Powell

Printed in the UK by
The King's Fund

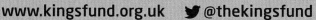

**The King's Fund** is an independent charity working to improve health and care in England. We help to shape policy and practice through research and analysis; develop individuals, teams and organisations; promote understanding of the health and social care system; and bring people together to learn, share knowledge and debate. Our vision is that the best possible care is available to all.

**www.kingsfund.org.uk**   **@thekingsfund**